How to Survive
and
Maybe Even Love
YOUR LIFE
AS A NURSE

How to Survive and Maybe Even Love YOUR LIFE AS A NURSE

KELLI S. DUNHAM, RN, BSN, and

STACI J. SMITH, RNC

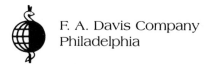

F. A. Davis Company
Philadelphia

4-06

F. A. Davis Company
1915 Arch Street
Philadelphia, PA 19103
www.fadavis.com

Copyright © 2005 by F. A. Davis Company

Printed in the United States of America

Last digit indicates print number: 10 9 8 7 6 5 4 3 2 1

Acquisitions Editor: Robert G. Martone
Developmental Editor: Alan Sorkowitz
Design Manager: Joan Wendt
Project Editor: Danielle J. Barsky

As new scientific information becomes available through basic and clinical research, recommended treatments and drug therapies undergo changes. The author(s) and publisher have done everything possible to make this book accurate, up to date, and in accord with accepted standards at the time of publication. The author(s), editors, and publisher are not responsible for errors or omissions or for consequences from application of the book, and make no warranty, expressed or implied, in regard to the contents of the book. Any practice described in this book should be applied by the reader in accordance with professional standards of care used in regard to the unique circumstances that may apply in each situation. The reader is advised always to check product information (package inserts) for changes and new information regarding dose and contraindications before administering any drug. Caution is especially urged when using new or infrequently ordered drugs.

Library of Congress Cataloging-in-Publication Data

Dunham, Kelli S.
  How to survive and maybe even love your life as a nurse / Kelli S. Dunham and Staci J. Smith.
    p. ; cm.
  Includes bibliographical references and index.
  ISBN 0-8036-1158-7 (alk. paper)
  1. Nursing—Vocational guidance. 2. Nurses—Job satisfaction.
  3. Nursing—Psychological aspects.
  [DNLM: 1. Nursing. 2. Career Mobility. WY 16 D917h 2005] I. Smith, Staci J.
II. Title.
  RT82.D86 2005
  610.73 '06' 9—dc22   2004027691

Introduction

Whether the ink is still wet on your license, or you've had the "RN" after name for decades, we want to start out by saying "congratulations" for all your success so far. You've probably had to overcome obstacles in your journey (if not, write and let us know how you managed this!) and yet, here you are. You're not only a nurse; we're guessing if you're taking the time to read this book you're also a proactive person, interested in making your nursing career and your life as a nurse the best that it can be.

We believe this book can help. Not because we're scholarly experts with multiple doctorate degrees in nursing philosophy and theory but because we talked with the real experts in making a success of a nursing, working RNs. We contacted hundreds of nurses (through nursing listservs and personal networks) and surveyed (okay, some might say "bugged") them about their experiences. Their advice is the substance of the majority of this book, although our experiences certainly informed the discussion and helped us frame the questions.

And without sounding too sentimental, we were gratified by the response. Nurses were eager to share their knowledge and we found that many of them, in fact, did love their lives as nurses.

Who Are We and Why Are We Writing This Book?

You undoubtedly know by now that we are the authors of this book, Kelli Dunham and Staci Smith. We're Philadelphia-based nurses with a passionate belief in the inherent capacity of each nurse to excel in today's challenging nursing environment.

Staci: Let me tell you about my co-author Kelli. Kelli is 36 years old. Before starting her formal nursing education, Kelli traveled the world attempting to satisfy a lifelong goal of helping those in need. Kelli graduated from Hahnemann University in 1998. When she graduated, she worked at a nurse-managed health center and now works with the Nurse-Family Partnership of Drexel University doing community outreach with first-time, high-risk moms. Kell is also the proud mom of *How to Survive and Maybe Even Love Nursing School*, the prequel to this book. Along with her full-time public health nursing job, Kelli also manages to work as a stand-up comedian, playing gigs throughout the country.

Kelli: Staci is a 20-year veteran of nursing. An RN at 19, she has worked in a number of different settings, including psych, labor and delivery, psychiatric managed care, in the SICU, MIC, telemetry, prison, and now in the ED. Staci has a unique, compassionate spirit and combines her professionalism and compassion in a nursing life that I believe is exemplary. Staci is also an accomplished writer and has a well-honed sense of humor. When it became obvious that I would want a nurse with extensive hospital experience to write this book with me, Staci was an obvious choice. In addition to her nursing career, Staci makes time for lots of involvement in community and women's concerns and is an accessible mom to her two teenage daughters.

Note, if you will, that we've called this book *How to Survive and Maybe Even Love Your Life as a Nurse* and those words were carefully chosen. To be a truly fulfilled person, it's not enough to love your work, although that's a good start. We believe it's important to have the skills to make your career enhance your life and your life enhance your career.

So how does one develop these skills? Well, experience, as the old saying goes, is the best teacher and many of the things in nursing (as in life) we just have to learn on our own. But life being as short as it is, it never hurts to benefit from other folks' experiences, which is what we are presenting in this book.

Since we know that readers may be coming at this subject with extensive experience, some experience, or none at all, we've tried to include information that will be helpful and interesting to nurses at all points in their careers. And because some people will undoubtedly need more information than we have room for, we've included comprehensive lists of resources to point you in a right direction to get this information.

It is our hope that different parts of this book will be helpful to you at different points in your career. We tried very hard to talk about the entire lifespan of a nursing career. Since increasing retention is one of the most important factors in decreasing the nursing shortage, we especially wanted to talk with nurses who have spent a lifetime as nurses and find out what their secrets are, and just as importantly, what they wish they had done differently.

We have both discovered that nursing is much more than a job; it becomes rather a part of your identity, and is reflected in the way you think and the way people think about you. We hope that this book will assist you as you grow into this role and accept both its negative and positive ramifications and to take your own place in the community of nursing.

So as you take your first peruse through this book, please (as the 12-steppers say) take what you want and leave the rest. Hopefully the irreverence of this book will be useful for some comic relief as well.

Thanks for taking this trip with us, and we hope that you can absorb some of the (to quote the 12-steppers again) experience, strength, and hope from your fellow nurses, and that this will help guide you through both the difficult and the great times ahead.

Acknowledgments

First of all, we'd like to heartily thank the many, many nurses who agreed to be interviewed for this book and who filled out our (extremely long) survey. Their patience and helpfulness showed real generosity toward their fellow nurses and proved, once again, that nurses do care about one another.

Especially helpful were the folks from Graduate Hospital and the 11th Street Family Health of Drexel University who permitted us to distribute the survey, as well as the very supportive Sally Dillon, nurse manager of the Graduate ED.

We'd also like to thank the amazing accountant Wally Moyer (www.thebottomlineinc.net) for allowing us to interview him for the financial planning part of Chapter 9.

In addition, Virginia Lindler (a great nurse as well as a meticulous fact checker) was instrumental in developing the Resources sections of each chapter.

Kelli especially wants to thank Maura, Beth, Wesley, and Viola as well as all the folks at the 11th Street Family Health Center of Drexel and the Greater Nurse Family Partnership community for their support and for providing a great place to work.

Staci especially wants to thank Donna Marie Opuszynski whose tolerance and understanding helped make this book possible as well as the amazing Cara and Jeanine Smith for their support and for being their mom's cheerleaders.

Contributors

Jen Borek, RN (ADN, 2003, Delaware County Community College)
Staff Nurse
Crozier Chester Medical Center
Chester, Pennsylvania

Maura C. Kelly, BS (1994, Temple University)
President
MCK Consulting
Philadelphia, Pennsylvania

Reviewers

Janine Anderson, RN, BSN
Broken Hill Base Hospital
Broken Hill, Australia

Hannah Burgess, RN, BSN
Children's Memorial Hospital
Chicago, Illinois

Sheria A. Hudson, RN, BSN
Christiana Care Health Services
Wilmington, Delaware

Anne Lamesse, RN, BScN, MScN, PHCNP
Nursing Professor
Fanshawe College, Health Sciences Division
London, Ontario, Canada

Michelle McMillion
Registered Nursing Student
Golden West College Huntington
Huntington, California

Rebecca Renner, RN, BSN
Pediatric ICU, University of Chicago
Chicago, Illinois

Neil Tassoni, RN, BSN, MA
University of Minnesota
Boynton Health Service
Minneapolis, Minnesota

Mike Vad, RN, BSN
Hennepin County Medical Center
Minneapolis, Minnesota

Contents

𝆑𝆑𝆑𝆑𝆑 **CHAPTER 7**

𝆑𝆑𝆑𝆑𝆑 **CHAPTER 8**

𝆑𝆑𝆑𝆑𝆑 **CHAPTER 9**

𝆑𝆑𝆑𝆑𝆑 **CHAPTER 10**

𝔊𝔊𝔊𝔊𝔊 CHAPTER 11

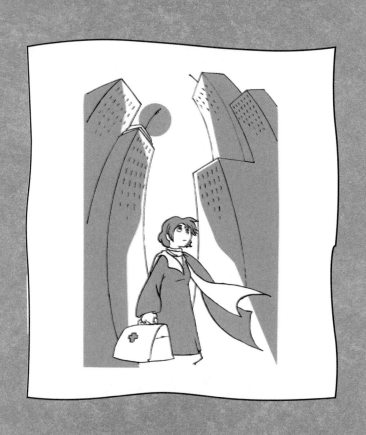

1

CHAPTER

After Nursing School: Now What? Taking Stock

A New Grad Speaks

"It's over? I'm really...a nurse? When did that happen?"

Craig Dean, RN

 ## The Nursing School Experience: What Did It Mean to You?

Guess what? You did it! You graduated from nursing school, passed the NCLEX, and now you have those oh-so-sweet little letters "RN" after your name. There had to be moments—perhaps many of them—when you wanted to throw in the towel, throw off your scrubs and run away from the whole, shall we say, "challenging" process. But you didn't. You persevered (perhaps with the assistance of sizeable amounts of coffee and/or chocolate) and here you sit with a smile on your face and a license in your hand.

But now what?

Well, you probably want to—as one new grad from Arkansas put it—"run off like a gazelle on crack" to start your job search. But whoa ....wait a minute. The nursing world is out there, yours for the taking, but it will be there tomorrow, too. Spend just a tiny moment in some well-deserved reflection.

If you've got one handy, peruse a picture of yourself taken at the very beginning of nursing school. If you've had the same college ID all through school, the photo on it is ideal. Aside from the loss of some substantial "bright-eyed-and-bushy-tailed"–ness that you displayed in

3

the photo, you probably don't look that much different now. Okay, you might have a few extra pounds on your frame, thanks to the amazing stress-busting effects of chocolate, and you might have a few (okay, a lot) more gray hairs. Nevertheless, that is still you, the same person who marched with enthusiasm into the bookstore to purchase your first stethoscope, who couldn't sleep the night before your first clinical rotation, and who got a not insignificant thrill when signing "SN" after your name for the first time.

In this time of transition, this knowledge should reassure you that you are that same person who had the drive and enthusiasm to get through nursing school. Remember this even as you acknowledge how nursing school has changed you. Some new grads, such as Jill Hall of California, are not going to be looking back fondly at their nursing school years any time soon. "[I found] nursing school a soul destroying experience," she said, "because of the demeaning attitude of some of the instructors and unreasonable requirements."

Some traditional college-age grads stated that even though they enjoyed their nursing school experience, they nevertheless felt slightly "ripped off." As one new grad said, "I don't need beer slides or wild keg parties, but it would have been nice to spend occasional time casually reading under an oak tree, instead of running off to clinical. At graduation, when we were lining up with our caps and gowns for graduation, I started feeling a little ticked off. I realized I hadn't been to college, I had been to nursing school." Other new grads with whom we talked literally bubbled with joy when describing their time at school. "I've been in the workforce for years," said a new grad for whom nursing was a second career. "But nursing school was the first really positive challenge I've had in a long time."

In general, we found that most new grads felt ambivalent about the time they spent in nursing school. Very recent new grads, especially, seemed to be literally reeling from conflicting feelings. They often felt very proud to finally have the RN after their name, but were anticipating reality shock as they prepared to transition to their new role.

Clearly, having conflicting thoughts and feelings at this point is normal.

So please, please, please, PLEASE try not to berate yourself if you feel slightly "burnt out" even though you've only just finished school. You are beginning the process of combining a working reality with an ideal that was presented to you in school. And remember, thanks to your clinical rotations, you've actually been out there in the trenches. You've experienced life as a nurse so you already know some of the challenges you will encounter in your profession. Because of this, at this point you may feel differently about your profession than your roommate feels about her paleontology program after spending four years perhaps writing papers and gazing at drawings of dinosaurs' navels and having little contact with flesh and blood paleontologists. Give your roommate a year and she'll be calling you with tales of woe from the bowels of the paleontology profession, or sending you e-mails that start, "Like the raptasaurus during the Neolithic period, paleontologists may not survive if we keep eating our young." Of course, you won't gloat, but it might give you a tinge of joy to read such an e-mail and remember that—in addition—Paleontology Pam will probably never in her career be offered a sign-on bonus. Of course, she'll probably also never learn what a "code brown" is or have to deal with projectile vomiting, but, after all, each job has its occupational hazards.

 Preparing for a Time of Transition

An important factor in making any transition is giving ourselves credit for what we've accomplished that got us to this point. In the case of the new grad, you've done the substantial work that finishing nursing school and passing the NCLEX requires, but you've also done much more.

Your nursing school experience didn't take place in a vacuum, you also worked hard to simultaneously manage all your other affairs. Perhaps you took care of kids, or held an outside job, or did volunteer work, or stayed active in your church. Or perhaps you did all of the above! Maybe you were a student who had been out of school for a long time and found that you needed extra tutoring to stay up with your classes. Even if you were a single, traditional-age student and you ate in the school cafeteria, you undoubtedly had to manage relationships with roommates, develop new friendships, and perhaps deal with the difficulty of being away from home the first time.

You may have overcome great obstacles to get into nursing school. If the whole nursing school shebang was harder because you have an unsupportive spouse, a learning disability, test anxiety, or even just a bad case of low self-esteem, give yourself credit for the work it took for you, especially, to get through.

Also, think about the myriad of little tasks you had to organize and complete just to make the nursing school experience happen! How many financial aid forms have you filled out? How many times have you washed your uniform? Touched up your sneakers with white shoe polish (or white nail polish in a pinch)?

The point of this is not to make you ruminate about all the energy that nursing school required, but to remind you of how organized, self-disciplined, and hard-working you have been. Goal-oriented people (which you probably are to some extent or you most likely wouldn't have gotten through school) sometimes reach a goal, only to sprint on toward the next goal with no break and no celebration.

Don't let that be you! You worked hard and you deserve accolades and celebration. The world being as it is, sometimes other folks in your life may not be able to figure out that you want those accolades, so, if necessary, provide them for yourself. If you haven't already had one, tell your friends, spouse, fishing buddies, or bridge partners to throw you a party, or throw one for yourself. If parties aren't your thing, ask a few close friends to go out to eat in celebration, or use your frequent flyer miles to take off for a sun-drenched destination. If you're really broke, go to the public library and check out a good book, preferably one that doesn't contain the words "diagnosis" or "paradigm," or make mention of Maslow's hierarchy of needs. Make popcorn and spend the day reading on the couch (or even in bed, because popcorn doesn't produce many crumbs).

The insecurity of not having a job yet often makes new grads want to do nothing but look for a job. But many of the experienced nurses we talked with said that they wished they had taken off some time between graduation and starting their career. While you may be spending time getting reacquainted with your spouse, friends, family, and children, and celebrating your successes, you might also want to spend some quality time with yourself and get back in touch with the idea of doing something...gasp...dare we say it, fun! For ideas, see the box, Refueling: Dates with the Other Side of Your Brain.

So we've made our case for throwing parties and such, but we also realize you are feeling the pinch of a new reality. The immediate new-grad period can be an exciting time, but it can be turbulent, too.

For example, many new grads found that partners and family members who were helpful through school may be frustrated by the new grad's inability to instantly resume their previous part of the housework, childcare, or income generation. Another new grad described a boyfriend who—although he was patient with her limitations on time and energy while she was in school—immediately started pushing for more commitment once she graduated.

Also, there may have been many things—both logistical and emotional—that you have had to delay dealing with until you were done with school. These could range from grieving over the loss of a family member to having bunion surgery to weeding through the

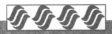

Refueling: Fun Dates with the Other Side of Your Brain

Read something that makes you laugh. Pick up the funny pages or a book by David Sedaris, Erma Bombeck, or Molly Ivins. There are quite a few of these available on CD or tape, so you can even listen to them while exercising or driving to job interviews. You can also check out some of the humor sites suggested in the Resources section for Chapter 3.

Go to a museum. Don't go to a medical museum, mind you, or some place where they keep nursing paraphernalia from years past. Find a real museum with paintings or dinosaur bones or stuffed buffalo. Maybe you'll even run into your paleontology-studying roommate (if so, buy her lunch, remember she's not going to get a sign-on bonus!)

Check out one of the higher-end video arcades that have the whole body movement virtual reality games. Virtual skiing, snowboarding, and jet skiing are all fun, but for good ol' frustration relief, don't miss virtual boxing. Pow!

Watch a movie. No, don't rent a movie so you can fold laundry and fix the kids' bikes while you watch it. Go to the theater, where it's just you, the popcorn, and perhaps someone you call Snugglebunny.

Go to an amusement park. Yes, it can be costly, but if you look for coupons (usually offered through fast-food places or on soft drink cans) you can save some cash and still have a great time. Ride the rollercoaster, drive the bumper cars, and make some noise on the carousel. Come on, you know you want to!

several thousand pieces of outgrown clothing your children have amassed in the past few years.

In addition, there may be situations in your life that have been bad for some time (e.g., fighting with a spouse or partner), but that you attributed to the stress of nursing school. If you've finished school and find that the situation continues to be bad, you may be forced to make difficult decisions at a time when you have little stability. You'll want to be careful about making too many changes at once, but at the same time, depending on your situation, you may find that finishing nursing school gives you the shot of confidence you need to make a long-needed change.

Even if you have been able to stay caught up on daily chores (let us know how you did that, okay?) and don't have a family or health crisis looming, you may still find yourself bothered by a feeling of generalized anxiety whenever you stop to catch your breath. The uncertainty of this time can be tough, so give yourself time and space to adjust. Check out some of the Websites and books in the Resources section of this chapter for tips on dealing with the stress of uncertainty. In addition, we've

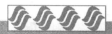

Journaling Idea: Taking Stock of Your Nursing School Experience

- What strengths have you discovered since you started school?
- Who has "been there" for you the past few years?
- What did you learn about your support system? About how easy or difficult it is for you to accept help? About how you handle stress?
- What activities did you eliminate in order to make time for school? Do you want to resume these activities? Is there anything else you might want to consider adding to or subtracting from your life now that you have had this experience?

included a journaling exercise that may help you start to sort out your thoughts and feelings about the past few years.

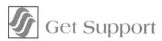

Get Support

So, you might be thinking, "How long until this starts feeling better?" And the answer is, it depends. It depends on your personal situation mostly, of course, and on how much emotional reserve you've been able to maintain to deal with the stress of change. But in addition, it depends on how well you use your support network.

You know...your support network, the folks who have been helping out while you were chasing after your RN? Picking up your kids from school if you ran late at clinical; stopping by your house or dorm with homemade cookies; people from whom never was heard a discouraging word. Remember? Oh, well, even if you've not had much of a support system up until now, it's not too late to start building one.

The most obvious and most important source of mutual support is other new grads. Jill Hall, who has worked in the pediatric ICU since her graduation 2 years ago, had this advice: "[now that you've graduated]...find a fellow new grad and touch base from time to time. I have coffee with a classmate about once a month. We work in completely different fields yet have so much in common. We have grown up, as nurses, together so our issues are the same. Those coffee dates are a lifesaver."

For the last few years, you've had a ready-made peer group in your classmates. No matter how glad you are to be rid of your classmates Patty Perfect and Sammy the Smart Alec, you may find yourself missing the camaraderie of the shared role of student nurse.

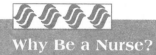

Why Be a Nurse?

Here is a list of reasons nursing students, new grads, and experienced nurses gave for picking the nursing profession:

- I want to make more money than I've done in the past.
- To help people.
- Because I want a transferable skill. I know I can go anywhere and find a job.
- To make a difference in sick kids' lives.
- To make enough money to leave my abusive husband.
- Because I know it will be a real challenge.
- To use my compassion and my smarts at the same time.
- Because when I was in the hospital after a car accident, I saw what nurses really do and started to admire the profession.
- Because of the flexibility. I can work night shift and always be there when my kids come home from school.
- Because nursing is a career where you are always learning something.
- For the excitement. I know no two work days are ever going to be the same.

So if you haven't been in contact with them already, put down this book (go ahead...we'll wait) and call some of your school chums to schedule a get-together. Go on!

In addition to staying in touch with friends you made in school, now is the time to reconnect with anyone who encouraged your nursing aspirations, particularly if that person is a nurse. Ask them to remind you why someone would want to be nurse in the first place. Write down what they say, add all your personal reasons, too (if you get stuck, see Why Be a Nurse?), make photocopies of the list and post them in some strategic places in your house (laminated in the shower perhaps?). Refer to them when you're feeling most uncertain.

Let Me into the Dressing Room, I Want to Try on My New Role

In addition to being full of personal turmoil, the immediate postgrad period can also be full of professional uncertainty.

At school you'd worked your way up from being a brand-new SN who perhaps struggled with everything from operating the side rails on your

9

patients' beds to learning the right way to use a fracture pan. When you graduated, you were probably a trusted part of the school/hospital team. Maybe you were even mentoring new students.

If you're working as a GN, you may find that while you were the top dog in school, you're back to being the lowest in the pack. In addition, even if you loved clinical rotations and your instructors let you do everything from juggling 10 patients to giving IV push meds to taking orders off charts, you may find that you still feel very unprepared to do what is expected of you in your new role. See A New Grad Speaks for the journal entries of Jen Borek, a May 2003 graduate of the ADN program at Delaware County Community College in Pennsylvania.

Some new nurses found it helpful to think of this transitional period as one more part of school. "A good nurse is always learning," said RA, who has worked as an RN for 10 years, "and the new grad period is a very intense learning time. Nursing schools can teach you how to think like a nurse, and act like a new a nurse, but it takes experience out in the real world to teach you how to really be a nurse."

In addition to the angst from your new role within the world of nursing, you may also be feeling pressured by the perceptions of nursing from the world at large. You may find that when you proudly share about your newly acquired "RN" title with everyone from the guy sitting next to you on the bus to your third cousin thrice removed, you get mixed reactions. Although studies have confirmed that the general public sees nurses as extremely trustworthy, there is also plenty of misinformation out there about what exactly nurses do.

It is far outside of the scope of this book to address the myriad of social and political circumstances that contribute to some of the lack of respect that the nursing profession is afforded, although we chat about it briefly in Chapter 11 as a contributing factor to the nursing shortage. Media portrayals of nursing (e.g., experienced emergency nurses on the television drama *ER* having to be told to take vital signs), the perception of nurses as "only caretakers," and the history of nursing as a female-dominated (and therefore lower status) occupation are just some of the factors that contribute to an often incomplete understanding of the role of nurses in health care.

Collectively, nurses can address some of the systemic problems that keep nursing from getting the respect it deserves (more on that in Chapter 11). Individually, nurses also have the capacity to help facilitate this type of change. As the nursing shortage has worsened, there has been a flurry of articles in nursing career magazines (invariably written by nurses who have not been involved in hands-on care in years) exhorting nurses to be a public relations force for the profession by

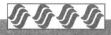

A New Grad Speaks

Night before orientation—Sunday, June 15, 2003
I feel like it's the night before first day of school. I have checked and re-checked my things a hundred times. Such decisions, what new scrubs to wear, etc. We are to report at 7:45 a.m. outside of the nursing office. Did I set the alarm? I'd better check again.

Monday, June 16, 2003
I arrived promptly at 7:30 outside the nursing office, I decided to give myself enough time to stop for coffee and I was still early. When I got there, there were a few other new grads waiting. By 7:45 the entire group of 11 girls was there. You have never seen such gleaming white shoes and crisp new uniforms. We were all taken into a classroom where we watched movie after movie. We were given a video overview of everything from fire safety to CPR to how to fill out an incident report. I was ready to crawl in bed by 11 a.m. After a long lunch we saw a few more videos and we were finished for the day.

Tuesday, June 17, 2003
New classroom, new set of movies. I never realized there was such a market for health training videos. I've decided if this whole nursing thing doesn't work out I may have an acting career in these movies. Mr. Jones, Mr. Jones... Are you alright? Call a code! Anyway in addition to the movies we were shown how to use the IV pumps. Finally a speaker from the Domestic Abuse Outreach program came to instruct us on our role in helping victims of abuse.

Wednesday, June 18, 2003
Hooray, first day on the floor. I was paired with Ellen, a nurse manager who floats in the hospital. We were assigned to 2E, a med-surg telemetry floor. This floor is primary care so we had 4 patients and gave them total care. Everything from vital signs to baths to meds. It was an exciting day; I really felt like a nurse.

Thursday, June 19, 2003
Today we were back in the classroom for speakers. We had representatives from all parts of the hospital in to speak to us. We had respiratory therapy, dietary, hospital safety, infection control, HR to go over insurances, occupa-tional health, PT to show us good body mechanics and someone who went over HIPPA regulations. It was an exhausting day.

Friday, June 20, 2003
Today I finished my first week on the floor with Ellen again. This time we were sent to 4S, a med-surg orthopedic floor. This floor is run differently than 2E, On 4S, there is a charge nurse, a meds nurse, and a mixture of LPNs and

(continued)

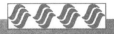
aides that provide the rest of the care. Ellen and I were responsible for giving meds to one side of the 36-bed unit. We listened to report, did chart checks and got started. We had meds to give at 7:30, 8, 9, 10, 11, 12, 1, and 2. Thank God for the 1-hour window. We gave the 7:30 insulins first, then we gave the 8s and 9s which were the bulk. At this point it was almost 10. We then gave the 10s, 11s, and 12s by around 12:15. We then took a much needed lunch, came back, did the 1s and the 2s by around 1:45. Then we had to write nursing notes for the aides we had assigned to us. Finally the day was over. I got home and collapsed, it was finally the weekend. Now the real fun begins. Did I really have this much laundry to do? Oh and don't forget to study for boards!

Monday, June 23, 2003

Just as my feet stopped aching from Friday, it was time for work again. Today Ellen and I are on 4S again passing meds. Today was much smoother. I was really in a routine. The day flew by. We even got to hang blood.

Tuesday, June 24, 2003

This is the day that I had been waiting for. Today I sat for the NCLEX. I decided to do it now figuring there is no reason to wait any longer. I felt as prepared as I could be. I took the Kaplan course, and did about 7500 questions over the last several months in preparation. This was it! The testing site was as secure as the Pentagon. You needed to bring your ATT (authorization to test) along with two forms of ID, one with a picture. We were warned that your name should be identical on all three to avoid any problem. I went in, took a number, and waited. I was then fingerprinted and had my picture taken. I was then led into the testing room where I was given a brief tutorial and then I began. I was so nervous! The machine shut off after 75 questions. I couldn't believe it was over. Now I had to wait. Either way today is my last day as a GN.

Wednesday, June 25, 2003

Today I was in a classroom again learning the hospital's computer system. It was an easy day putting in orders and looking up lab reports.

Thursday, June 26, 2003

Today I was back on the floor. I was on 2E again doing primary care. I had 4 patients and provided total care. It was a good day. As I was waiting for report to finish, I decided to check my messages on one of the phones at the nurses' station. It was then I heard the words Congratulations RN! from a friend (also a nurse) who had checked the Web to see if my license was issued. I passed! I can't believe I'm an RN! I almost fell out of my chair!

Friday, June 27, 2003

Today was my first day as an RN. I was on 2E, primary care. I had 6 patients, I ran around all day long. It was great. I hope I still feel this way in 30 years.

always talking positively about nursing, encouraging friends and relatives to consider nursing as a career, etc. We agree with these suggestions, but think they should be tempered with realism. As a new grad, you have energy and enthusiasm for the profession, and sharing that with folks will go a long way toward creating an understanding of, and promoting, nursing.

At the same time, there is a reason nurses have developed "gallows humor" to an art form and created such colorful terms as "circling the drain." Ours is a challenging occupation, and to pretend otherwise seems disingenuous. Being a nurse can be extremely rewarding (we think so or we wouldn't have suggested in the title that you can love your life as a nurse), but we don't need to Pollyanna-ize the profession or take the entire burden of reversing the nursing shortage on ourselves. If we are positive examples, nursing will sell itself.

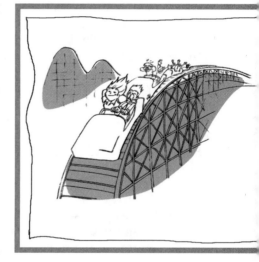

As you start your new career, and while you (hopefully) have a few free minutes, you may want to put aside some reading material that reminds you of the ideals of nursing. Some suggestions are listed in the Resource section at the end of this chapter and include biographies of accomplished nurses, collections of touching or inspiring stories related by nurses, etc. When you have a horrendous day on the floor and want to come home and start an extra-large bonfire using your scrubs, drug guide, and this book as kindling, you can instead put your feet up, sip a cup of tea, and by reading, re-inspire yourself. You'll feel better, and your neighbors won't have to summon the fire marshal.

The Year of Med/Surg Experience Debate

Ah, the beloved controversy: do new grads need to do a year of med/surg nursing or not? Like many of the new grads and experienced nurses we talked with, we have differing perspectives on this. One of the authors (Kelli) bypassed the med/surg year and instead went directly from school to an RN position at a nurse-run primary care clinic. After nursing school, Staci worked as a labor and delivery nurse on the unit where she had been a tech during school. She became interested in psych nursing and realized she could not get a psych nurse position without doing the med/surg year. She changed to a nearby community hospital where she did med/surg for a year, and found it very challenging but essential to her nursing career because she learned every organizational skill she needed there. Both of us felt the choices were best for our careers.

There are benefits and drawbacks for both sides of the controversy, and we've summarized them in the box that follows. Perhaps Lourdes Rodriguez, a Philadelphia-based nurse who has been practicing for more than 20 years in a variety of settings, summarized the thoughts of most of the nurses we talked with when she said, "It depends on the nurse's goals and what she feels is appropriate for the situation." Once you carefully weigh the pros and cons, it will become clear what choice will serve you best in your aspirations and which will be the best for the patients you will serve.

Before we leave this topic, however, we wanted to point out that your choice does not necessarily have to be an either/or proposition. With some creativity, nurses can take action to mitigate the negative consequences of either choice. For example, a nurse who goes directly to the ICU can help supplement her or his knowledge base and feel more comfortable on the unit by studying during off hours. A nurse who feels strongly about wanting to enter a specialty field as soon as possible but still wants time to develop skills on the med/surg floor can arrange with the hospital to work 6 months on med/surg and then transfer to another unit. A new grad interested in OB might ask to work part-time on the labor floor and part-time on a med/surg floor (hey, there's a nursing shortage going on, it never hurts to ask).

Setting Your Preliminary Career Goals

We can almost hear the nurses out there in reader-land saying, "Okay, now that we've had some fun, thrown a party, buddied up with another new grad, and journaled about the anxiety of this transitional time, NOW is it finally time to look for a job?"

Yes. Well, um okay, almost. Go ahead, read the next chapter and start sending out your resume.

But before you start distributing it willy nilly (whatever that means), take a moment and consider this: what is the single most important

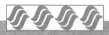

Pros	Cons
The year of med/surg experience is really the completion of nursing school education and is needed if new grads are ever going to feel confident in their nursing abilities.	Spending a year on the med/surg floor for nurses who are not interested in hospital nursing is a waste of nurses' and facilities' time.
Nursing school doesn't give enough experience in basic skills, especially assessment skills for new grads to practice safely in specialty areas.	Assessment skills, especially, are specialized. What a new grad learns on a med/surg unit will only be somewhat helpful in a public health or community setting. A nurse's time is better used in the concentration area.
Med/surg year allows new grad time to learn valuable skills like leadership, dealing with docs, time management, and on-the-spot emergency management that can't be learned in school.	These skills can be learned in more specialized settings as well, and the nurse will be more motivated to learn them in an area of interest.
The med/surg year is a commonly accepted part of the "dues paying" process of entering a new profession. New grads who don't do a year of med/surg nursing will not be as respected as "real nurses" by their colleagues.	The first year in a new profession is always arduous. Instead of thinking in terms of "paying dues," a more suitable model might be rewarding nurses for entering the profession by allowing them to choose an area of interest and providing support for them in the form of extensive orientation, ongoing education, and supportive preceptorships.
Wider variety of patients.	Learning one area of care well.

characteristic you are looking for in a job? For example, maybe you want a job with flexibility to spend more time with your kids. Maybe your first priority is making lots of cash so you can get your student loans paid off. Maybe you want a job that will enable you to move back to Montana to take care of your Aunt Mona. There are many other possibilities also. New grads we talked with had various top priorities when looking for their first job, including being close to home to have a short commute, having a nurse manager who was sympathetic to new grads, finding an institution with a strong precepting program, being able to work in a particular specialty area, not having to work night shift, working with a particular patient population, avoiding a particular patient population ("I know I can't work with older folks," said one nurse, "they drive me crazy."), and finding an institution that had liberal continuing education benefits.

Of course, in some areas and in some parts of the nursing shortage swing cycle, you may have to start with time on a med/surg floor, or you won't be able to get another type of job. Clearly in this situation your top priority is finding a med/surg unit that will take you. If this is not your current situation, you may very well have no idea what your top priority is (said one new grad, "It's all important!"). In this case, skip ahead to Chapter 4, "Considering Opportunities," and look at the lists of options available to help you decide.

A tip—at this point, one of the things you might be doing is eliminating as potential choices any situations that you know will make you miserable. Don't feel guilty about this, a lot of lives could be made much better if people followed their instincts about this. For example, one of us (Kelli) is very sensitive to light variations and needs a lot of sunlight and fresh air to feel happy. Working as a home visiting nurse is a good choice for her, but working night shift in a cave-based nursing home in the Alaskan wilderness would not be. On the other hand, for some nurses, a job working in such a nursing home might be a dream come true. The key is to pay attention to your real needs and wants, not what you think you should need or want. A nurse recruiter may tell you they're "desperate" for nurses on her hospital's pediatric oncology unit. But if you take the job even though the idea of working with really sick kids makes you almost ill with sorrow, then pretty soon it's you who is going to be desperate to get a new job.

At this point in your pre-job search preparations, your research can take various forms. Some nurses choose to peruse the classified ads (links for online classifieds can be found in Chapter 3's Resource section) to see what kind of opportunities exist, other new grads use nursing-specific employment Websites or talk with nurses they know to learn the same thing. In addition, you may be getting calls—tons of them—from nurse recruiters (one recent grad said, "we refer to 'em as nurse-stalkers at my school") and if you don't mind the fact that they call you while you're eating dinner, they can be a valuable source of information. Ask lots of questions about what their institution has available, take lots of notes, and use the information for comparison when inquiring about other jobs.

Finally, take lots of deep breaths and keep things in perspective. Nurses are often the sort of folks who feel most comfortable with a well-defined plan, and a back-up plan, and back-up plans of their back-up plans and ba..., well, you get the picture. Nevertheless, you are not deciding right now what you are going to do for the rest of your life, only what you are going to do for the next year or so. Although nurse recruiters certainly wish it were otherwise, the average nurse we talked with stayed at a new-grad job for less than 18 months. It wouldn't be impossible for you to fall madly in love with the first place you choose to work and want to settle down there until you retire. On the other hand, you are making the best choice you can now with the information you have, and in a year you will have much more information

Resources

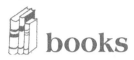 books

Bold, Laurence G. (1999).
Zen and the Art of Making a Living. New York: Penguin USA.

Billing itself as a "career guide for human beings" (as opposed to human "doings"), this huge tome might also be called the career guide for folks with a great deal of time on their hands. However, if you do have time, and don't mind some of the new age-y sounding terminology it uses (e.g., one chapter is called "vision questing"), this book can help you think about what you really want out of life, as opposed to what the dominant culture says you should want. It includes some practical tools, such as our favorite, the "playing-the-game" skills list.

Johnson, Spencer (1998).
Who Moved My Cheese. New York, New York:
G.P. Putnam's Sons.

This book is about two mice, named Sniff and Scurry, and two people named Hem and Haw. And, well, you might want to just read it yourself. Corny or not, this book has caught on because it addresses such a basic human problem—our difficulty in dealing with change.

Robbins, Alexandra (2001).
Quarterlife Crisis: The Unique Challenges of Life in Your Twenties. New York, New York: Tarcher/Putnam.

Ever heard of a quarterlife crisis? Probably not, but that doesn't mean you didn't have one, or aren't having one right now. If you—like many other new grads—are in your twenties, do yourself a favor and read this book. The author's research reveals there might be perfectly good reasons for feeling unsettled, stressed, anxious, and depressed at this time of your life, and that the proverbial light at the end of the proverbial tunnel is not—in fact—a proverbial train.

Thieman, Leann (2001).
Chicken Soup for the Nurse's Soul: 101 Stories to Celebrate, Honor and Inspire the Nursing Profession. Deerfield Beach, FL: Health Communications.

Despite the exponential (and somewhat clichéd) proliferation of the some kind of food for some kind of soul (we're waiting for "Tuna Fish for the Cat's Soul" ourselves) books, this tome is still destined to be a classic in nurse inspirational literature (okay, we just made up the genre). Great for boosting morale after a difficult 12-hour shift; don't miss the story called "Working Christmas Day." Also available on CD.

Van Betten, Patricia (2004).
Nursing Illuminations: A Book of Days. St. Louis, Missouri: Mosby.

A beautiful and interesting—if decidedly hard to lift because of its weight—book. It aims to illustrate the similarities and bonds between nurses from the past and nurses from the present in a collection of contributions from 366 nurses throughout history. Again, quite inspirational.

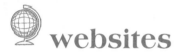 # websites

Discover Nursing
www.discovernursing.com
Yes, we know you've already discovered nursing or you wouldn't even be reading this book, but on those days when you need to rediscover nursing (i.e., when you're thinking "Why on earth am I doing this?"), surf on over to this site for some reminders. You can also order—for free—those stylin' "Because I'm a Nurse" posters to help with your personal recruitment efforts.

The Florence Nightingale Museum
www.florence-nightingale.co.uk/index.htm
If you ever find yourself in London (or if you live there), don't miss an opportunity to visit the Florence Nightingale Museum. The Museum houses an extensive collection of Florence Nightingale artifacts (including many of the more than 8000 letters she wrote in her lifetime), material connected with the Crimean War, and various objects connected with the Nightingale School and St. Thomas' Hospital (1860–1910). You can also watch a multimedia show about Florence Nightingale. If you go on a weekday when no school groups are scheduled, you just might have the place to yourself, and the museum staff (many volunteers, many retired nurses) will be extraordinarily pleased to answer any questions you might have. Very, very inspirational; nurses are known to shed tears here (don't say we didn't warn you!) Not going to England anytime soon? Check out the Website, where you can see pictures of some of the Museum's artifacts and read about the less well-known efforts of the "Lady with the Lamp."

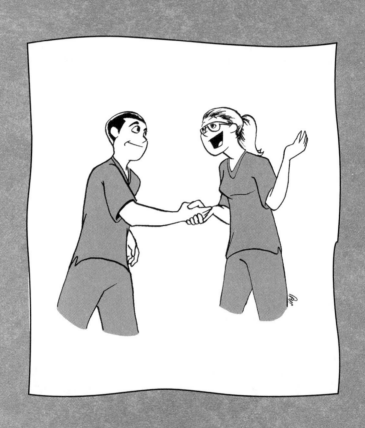

2

CHAPTER

Job Search Workout

A Nurse Speaks

"When I first got out of school, there was a nursing shortage sort of like now, but without the influence of HMOs, etc. The labor and delivery/postpartum/well baby nursery unit where I was employed as a nurse's aide while I was in school not only guaranteed me a job when I finished, but in retrospect, stopped only shy of coercing me into accepting! At 19, I was flattered and readily accepted their strong proposals. This landed me a nightshift position with little to no peer support, and experience a-plenty, but not in the field(s) I wanted to pursue. After about a year and a half, I found myself still in need of the med-surg experience. That was mandatory at the time for following a psych or critical care path (my two areas of interest). I still recall the nursery fondly but wish I had more foresight at the time. Then, I would have done a thorough search of the opportunities out there and not jumped at the first offer."

Layota Marshall, RN, Willow Run, Wisconsin

 Deciding What's Important to You

If you've been out of nursing for a while, are reentering the field and have some work experience under your belt, you may have a clearer picture of the area of nursing in which you now want to be employed. You may have vivid, fond memories of your psychiatric home health adventures or the intense nights you spent in that Bronx E.R. Maybe you're a new grad and you remember the thrill of precise, meticulous ostomy care (did you know there's a specialty in this field?) and you can see yourself doing nothing but this in your professional

1

capacity. If the above statements are true, congratulations. You've already started on the path toward one of most difficult decisions a working nurse must make: What specialty do I want to be involved with?

Many of us have a less clear concept of where we want to be. Many of us know what we don't want, but even those parameters can be lurking around in our heads formed in nebulous, fear-based packages. What's a nurse to do? The first thing is to tell yourself that you deserve to work in an area that will feel rewarding, important, and interesting to you. Then remind yourself that you have much to offer a prospective employer (this is true no matter what background you're coming from).

You can start the specialty selection process by creating a list that includes all the specialty areas you may want to consider. Even if it requires an advanced degree for a particular specialty area, write it down. After each area you list, make a note of what it is about that specialty area that really interests you and if you think you'd like to try a specialty area but feel overwhelmed by the idea, be honest and write that down, too. After you've done this, go back and prioritize this list (most favored to least favored; most feared to least feared; and so on). You may start to notice some trends or repeated themes in the areas you do or do not find interesting. This will give a sense of direction to your job search. You can begin to form goals about future specialty and/or education needs, if applicable, as well.

What should you do if you feel really at a loss about what specialty area interests you? We suggest going to your local bookstore conglomerate (or better yet, your local mom-pop book boutique) and get a couple of workbooks on personality testing, workplace temperaments, and so on (see the Resources section for this chapter for some ideas). Don't balk! This career thing will be taking up a lot of time in your life for a major portion of your life. It—and you—deserve some specific soul-searching investment.

It may be that you don't know what type of nursing will be most satisfying to you because you never really thought about what makes you smile or thrill or feel satisfied. Are you the quiet bookish type? Do you love the sound of a closing deal? Does delving deep into others' psyche make you deliriously happy? Can you find peace along with a hospice patient? Nursing has many different paths. There are as many specialties as there are personality types, or close to it. Remember, you deserve to do what feels most right for you. It has also been shown that if one is involved in work that one really resonates with, one does a better, more productive, enthusiastic job. Your patients, coworkers, and your managers will recognize and appreciate this more than you can imagine.

In addition, you will be guarding against burnout, another important consideration.

While you are working on your list of desired specialty areas, if you do notice a trend toward a lot of fear-based limits, think about why this is so. Staci likes to mantra in times of crisis (in a voice with varying degrees of earnestness or sarcasm depending on the specific crisis) a saying she once read, "Nothing nurtures success like a steadiness of purpose." It is invariably true that almost anything is possible with tenacious perseverance. This is true for a 92-year-old woman who climbed mount Everest (really happened), runners who run without legs, 60-year-olds who learn a second language, and nurses who want more than anything to become midwives or OR nurses but don't think they have what it takes. Do not rule out a career path that you really crave. Remember, you will be best at something you love and worked hard for, not something you settled for.

 ## Considering Fields of Practice

If you don't have a specialty area in mind, there certainly are plenty to consider. To get you thinking, we've included a brief list of some of the more popular nursing areas, including those you may not have been exposed to in nursing school. You can peruse the list then get more information about each of them (as well as many, many more) through the associations and Websites listed in the Resources section.

Critical Care Nurse

In this specialty, nurses are dealing (every day, all the time) with life-threatening health problems. Because of advances in health care, caring for very ill patients has become more and more complex, and a special, sometimes technically advanced, knowledge base is necessary for the best patient care and outcome. This is where a critical care nurse comes in. If you become a critical care nurse, the certification for critical care (CCRN) is a highly valued asset that employers often look for. The subspecialties for critical care nurses include adult, pediatric, and neonatal. Critical care nurses work with patients in a variety of settings, including adult and pediatric ICUs (intensive care units), neonatal ICUs, cardiac catheter labs, progressive care units, emergency departments, and increasingly, in home health settings, nursing schools, outpatient surgery centers, and flight units. Critical care RNs should desire to work with the most severely ill patient populations, many with multiple diagnoses. If you're going to be critical care nurse, you should be interested in working with medical technology (if Palm Pilots scare you, this might not be your field) and should desire to maintain continuing education and credentialing related to rapidly changing nursing and medical advances.

Emergency Nurse

The emergency nurse specializes in rapid assessment and triage of illness. Scenarios an emergency RN might encounter range from a child's midnight earache to cardiac arrest to MVA trauma. Both a general and specific knowledge base is necessary and developed with training and experience. There are two certifications related to emergency nursing: The CEN (certified emergency nurse) certification, and the TNCC (trauma nurse critical care) certification. Emergency nurses should also possess, or through their employer, work toward maintaining ACLS (advanced cardiac life support) and PALS (pediatric advanced life support) credentialing. Emergency RNs can work in many settings including emergency departments (pediatric, trauma centers, etc.), urgent care centers, schools/universities, prehospital transport, including airplane and helicopter transport, poison control centers, the military, telephone triage centers, crisis intervention centers, and even prisons, and, yes, cruise ships. The emergency RN should be interested in working in a fast-paced, constantly changing environment. As in critical care nursing, an emergency RN will need continuing education to maintain competence in current procedures and skills.

Hospice/Palliative Care Nurse

The focus of hospice nursing is providing comprehensive physical, psychosocial, emotional, and spiritual care to terminally ill patients and their families. Palliative care is utilized to ease suffering, control symptoms, and restore functional capacity when possible. The hospice/palliative nurse focuses completely on end-of-life issues and care. The career of a hospice nurse might include some working on-call (so that a nurse is available to the patient and family at all times), home or long-term facility visits, pain management, supportive physical care, and collaboration with a wide range of professional and volunteer persons (clergy, "meals-on-wheels," counselors, family members, social workers, etc.). A hospice RN should be able to focus on spiritual and existential issues that will arise for patients and their families while assisting them with comfort and physical needs. Certification is available (CHPN—Certified hospice/palliative nurse). If an RN has expert listening skills, paired with excellent pain management abilities and the ability to provide compassionate counseling, the RN can help promote a very high quality of life for the dying patient and his or her family.

Nurse Anesthetist

Certified registered nurse anesthetists (CRNAs) are the sole anesthesia providers in many hospitals in the United States and are directly reimbursed under the Medicare program. CRNAs begin with a bachelor's degree in nursing and continue with a master's degree in nurse anesthesia. A PhD is also available. Certification via a national exam is then completed and the anesthetist must recertify every 2 years. CRNAs are legally qualified to make independent judgments related to all aspects of anesthesia care. CRNAs may practice in hospital surgical suites, obstetrical delivery rooms, dental offices, podiatrist offices, ambulatory surgical centers, military facilities, and public health service facilities.

Nurse anesthetists, because of their advanced degrees, high level autonomy and its ensuing load of responsibility, command some of the highest levels of pay in the nursing arena. The percentage of CRNAs who are male is much higher than in the nursing profession as a whole.

Perioperative (OR) Nurse

Perioperative RNs assess, plan, and implement care for the surgical patient before, during, and after surgery. Creation and maintenance of a sterile environment during procedures and monitoring of the patient's physical well-being and stability throughout the surgical care continuum also factor in. A few specific intrasurgical positions for the RN include: scrub nurse, works within sterile field, assists surgeons, passes/handles instruments; circulating nurse, works outside of sterile field, manages OR environment and coordinates nursing team; RN first assistant, after additional training and experience, this RN may directly assist the surgeon with control of bleeding at the operative site, wound exposure, and suturing.

Perioperative nurses may also work in various administrative capacities related to OR budgeting, staffing, etc. Surgical subspecialties include: neurosurgery, cardiac surgery, trauma, pediatrics, oncology, general surgery, urology, ophthalmology, otorhinolaryngology (ear, nose, and throat), dental, plastic and reconstructive, and orthopedic.

OR nurses generally come from critical care or ER backgrounds where split-second assessment and decision making skills can be honed. The CNOR is the certification available to demonstrate advanced proficiency in the OR field.

Nurse Executive

Nurses work at various administrative levels, from nurse-manager of a unit to the chief nursing officer (CNO) of a hospital or network of hospitals. These networks can be based in acute care, ambulatory, or long-term care facilities. Nurse executives can work in the insurance industry, for a pharmaceutical organization, or within nursing unions or associations. Nurse executives help design plans for optimal, cost-effective patient care, partner with community and consumer groups to coordinate client/local population needs, facilitate interactions between medical, administrative, and nursing disciplines, and coordinate outcomes management via promotion of quality improvement and care systems implementation. Nurse executives also serve as role models and mentors to their staff and must have exquisite communication and diplomacy skills. Ideally they are advocates for nurses and the professionalism of nursing. They must maintain current licensure and ongoing education. A master's degree in nursing, hospital, or business administration is necessary, and strong leadership and management skills are preferably developed from experience in their chosen arena. Many CNOs have gone on to doctoral level education, with the FAAN (Fellowship of the American Academy of Nursing) a further mark of distinction and expertise at the highest level of nursing education.

Neonatal Nurse

Neonatal nurses work in specialized nurseries with infants during the first 28 days of life. Neonatal nurses work in level one, two, or three nurseries. Level one, or healthy newborn nurseries are quite rare now because of very short postpartum stays and rooming-in policies. Neonatal nurses do work with newborns and their mothers in this capacity. Level two nurseries provide specialty care for infants with medical issues ranging from illnesses to prematurity. Specialized feedings, intravenous supplementation, oxygen, and other modalities may be implemented. Level three, or neonatal intensive care, nurseries care for the neonate who needs the highest level of supportive technological care. This may include surgical interventions, ventilator support, and other modalities.

At the entry level, most institutions prefer to hire perspective neonatal nurses who have some experience in med-surg care, but depending on the status of the nursing shortage in your area and the availability of qualified staff, hospitals may be willing to train motivated nurses, even graduate or new RNs. This is true for many specialty venues. After experience in the NICU, further credentialing as a master's prepared neonatal nurse practitioner or clinical specialist is an option.

Labor and Delivery Nurse

L&D nurses care for women and their newborns during the antepartum, intrapartum, and postpartum phases of childbirth. This care occurs in the labor and delivery suite as well as in the postpartum unit, birthing centers, clinics, and physicians' offices. L&D nurses must combine empathy, holistic nursing practice, and patient education techniques with a high level of clinical expertise and prioritizing skills. L&D nursing can be highly rewarding within the context of a fast-paced, sometimes stressful environment. Specialty certification exams can be attempted after 2 years of practice. These specialty areas include: intrapartum nursing; postpartum nursing; and fetal monitoring

Psychiatric–Mental Health Nurse

Although all nurses—no matter what their specialty—must take into account the psychosocial needs of their patients throughout the care continuum, mental health nurses have these needs as their primary focus. Psych RNs work in various environments, such as inpatient and outpatient settings, home-care, community centers, military, crisis intervention centers, private practices, schools, prisons, and more. RNs may work with groups, individuals, or families. Mental health/competency assessments, therapy/group facilitation, assistance with coping and daily living skills, case management, monitoring and administration of psychobiological treatment regimens are all possible responsibilities a psych/mental health nurse may have.

Advanced practice RNs (psychiatric nurse practitioners and psychiatric mental health clinical nurse specialists) may work in the adult, geriatric, child, or adolescent mental health fields. They have the authority to provide a full range of primary mental health care services and counseling. In some states, advanced practice mental health RNs are able to prescribe medications.

School Nurse

The primary focus of a school nurse is to promote learning. This is accomplished by working to protect student and staff health and safety. School nurses must be familiar with both pediatric and mental health nursing. They serve as the health services coordinator for their school and are responsible for facilitating health education on topics as varied as sport safety, tobacco, alcohol and drug education, and STD and pregnancy prevention. School RNs provide injury/illness assessment, medication administration and assist in crisis interventions. They need strong diplomacy and communication skills as well as an ability to work independently, which may include performing in a liaison capacity between families, community, and children. School nurses also work with the population of mainstreamed children affected by physical and mental challenges. Further nursing assessments for these children's special needs, as well as possible nursing treatments (i.e., gastrostomy tube feedings, urine catheterization, tracheostomy care, etc.) are also under the school nurse's domain. To work as a school nurse, most states require that RNs have school nurse certification through the department of education or health. National certification is also available. The National Association of School Nurses recommends that all school nurses have a minimum of a baccalaureate degree and school nurse certification.

What we included here is definitely not an exhaustive list. This list does not even mention the entrepreneurial nurses who have built their own niches (book writing nurses, for instance). It should also be mentioned that experience in one area of nursing is always beneficial when entering another. Even when you change specialties, no skills become useless or lost. Every technique learned, every crisis diverted, every psychosocial or cultural nuance fathomed is another note—so to speak—in your repertoire. All experience makes you a better nurse, so don't be afraid you'll be "wasting time" trying different specialties. For instance, Staci's 6 years of psychiatric nursing have proven invaluable in the managed-care and ER units she has worked in since, and conversely, the ICU work done before her psych experience helped her build her assessment skills in the mental health field. Kelli's work in urban clinics with underserved populations made her exceptionally familiar with the pitfalls, illnesses, and issues her present clients (teenage mothers) face. The only constraints on the field you pursue should be ones dictated by your heart and your interests. C'mon, go for it!

Conducting Informational Interviews

So now you've narrowed it down to one or two possible areas of interest. Although you've done some thinking about it while you were reading Chapter 1 (and undoubtedly starting way, way, way before that), your next step can be to begin gathering firsthand information about possible places of employment and specialty areas. Think about the area hospitals, outpatient facilities, etc., you are interested in and, yes, make a list of these possible employment opportunities. Add to the list names of nurses you know who are involved in the specialty areas you're interested in. Also add to your list the local chapters of the professional organizations governing the specialty areas you are interested in (you can usually find them in the organization's Website).

With the ink barely dry on your list, it's time to go on some interviews. "But wait," you say, "I haven't finished my resume, I don't know what to look for, I don't know what to ask!" Well, we're not talking about a job interview, we're talking about informational interview. They take some time and work, but conducting successful informational interviews can really help make you a very hot commodity in your work field.

An informational interview is, well, an interview in which you seek (no surprises here) information. Also called "research" interviews, you can conduct informational interviews for a number of reasons, such as exploring and clarifying career goals, discovering unique or unadvertised job possibilities, expanding a professional network, accessing the most up-to-date career information, and identifying professional strengths and weaknesses.

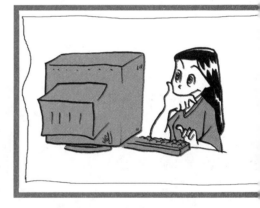

To prepare for an informational interview read about the field you're interested in and read any information available about the institution you'll be visiting (usually obtainable at the place itself, as well as the library, online, etc.) If it's a specific person or nurse you'll be meeting with, knowledge about his or her field will be sufficient. Prepare a list of questions to ask. Be prepared to go off the list when appropriate, but you'll be more comfortable and you'll get more practical information with a well thought out list of queries/concerns.

Then call the people and organizations you've identified. Letters can also be an acceptable way to make contact, but should be followed up with a phone call to make the appointment. Don't forget, this can be a nurse-manager of a unit you're interested in or this can be your best friend's 20-year veteran nurse aunt. Don't forget that people love to talk about the things they do and most people will greatly appreciate your motivation and interest in something so near to their heart and lives. Keep the interview to approximately one-half hour or slightly less for politeness' sake. Do dress appropriately and take notes through the interview. Remember, at this juncture, you're the interviewer! Before you leave, ask your contact to suggest names of others who might be helpful to you in your quest. In addition, be sure to request permission to use your interviewee's name when contacting these new resources.

Definitely send a written thank you note (within 1 week) to anyone you've interviewed. Compile all of your information. Adjust your job search and possibly your resume as a result of what you learn.

"So, what to ask?" we hear you say. Your questions, of course, should reflect your specific concerns and the specific specialty, but some ideas to get you started are included in the box What Do I Ask Now? Suggested Questions for Informational Interviews.

The process of conducting informational interviews will hopefully leave you feeling very prepared about the direction you want to go. You'll feel ready for employment interviews and these research interviews may have already opened up employment opportunities. They will also give you a very clear picture of your marketability, which leads us to our next section.

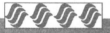

What Do I Ask Now? Suggested Questions for Informational Interviews

1. Beyond an RN, what training, certifications, etc., are required for this specialty?
2. What do you feel is the most satisfying aspect of working in this specialty area? What is the most challenging?
3. What is a typical day like working in this specialty?
4. What do you think are the most important personal qualities or abilities for someone who wants to work in this nursing specialty?
5. What is the demand like for nurses in this specialty area? Is this likely to change over the next few years or within this decade?
6. Are there any specialty organizations, Websites, listservs, professional journals, etc., that I should check out that would help me learn more about this specialty area?
7. What do you think about the experience level in terms of entering this specialty area (you can also ask "right out of school" if that is the case for you)?
8. (Once you've told the interviewer about your education, skills, experience, and interests) Can you think of any other specialty areas I should research before I make a final decision about my first job?
9. Is there anyone else I should talk to about this specialty area?

Inventorying Your Marketability

At this point, you have compiled a likes and dislikes list, you've read about the specialties you're interested in, and done your informational interviews. All of this should give an idea of the basic job requirements for your desired areas as well as some clues to the personalities that would do best in these areas. You may have even (hopefully) honed-down your "I want to do this type of nursing now" list to one or two ideas.

Now that the professionals you've interviewed have given you some real-life tips about what's important in your field of choice, you're ready to write (or possibly spruce up) that resume and take stock of your experience, your skills, and your education.

The first consideration is do you meet the basic requirements for your area of choice? If not, is this something that you are able to remedy now, or will this be a goal for future plans, after you've begun to work? If you've got the basics down, but don't have much relevant experience, think about possible ways to develop the attributes the profession is looking for in other venues (i.e., transferable skills). Motherhood can be a great aid in developing organizational and prioritizing abilities. Many non-nursing jobs require fast decision making skills. Think about community organizations, etc., that you've been involved with where your leadership qualities were fine-tuned.

If you're brand spanking new to the world of work, you are still bringing strength to the workplace. You have a fresh outlook and will be eager to make use of the many possibilities for training. You are certainly not jaded or prejudiced in any way toward unit organization, new treatment modalities, etc., so you are completely able to accept the mission and goals of your new employer wholeheartedly and as your own. The concept is to see your history as a worker and as a human in a positive light and convey that sense of your self to your desired employer.

Your desire for further educational pursuits is also a marketable commodity. Employers feel this is a mark of professionalism and loyalty to nursing and/or the chosen field of study. It conveys that you're in it for the long run. This loyalty may translate to "long-term employee" (for the institution that possibly will be reimbursing the college tuition), something that the nursing field values. As you advance your degree, you will also be a burgeoning asset and resource for your company. Find out what certifications are available in your chosen field and, if applicable, mention your desire to pursue certification at the appropriate time(s). Again, this reinforces to your prospective employer your commitment to professional excellence.

Many specialty areas do request and prefer that RNs applying for their positions have experience in their field or, let's say, in med-surg for a year. These rules are relaxed or even eradicated at times when need is high. During the time this book was written, the nursing shortage was raging. Couple this with new laws (in California) about mandated nurse/patient ratios and the graying of the nursing workforce, etc., and you had a very wide-open market. Many facilities were willing to take new RNs or even GNs into specialty areas and train them from the ground up. A lot of relaxation of the "year in med-surg" clause occurred, to the joy and chagrin of various camps. In this environment, it behooves you to attempt to get your foot in the door exactly where you want to be. If you're turned down because of inexperience, you will at least be able to ascertain exactly what they need and work toward those goals. Don't forget to use the contacts you made while doing your informational interviewing. It increases your chances of success exponentially when people feel they know you, or you have someone that can vouch for your character to the hiring staff person.

You've taken stock and now it's time to put all this dynamic and positive information into a tidy little format. Hence....

Preparing a Resume and Cover Letter

Your Resume

Although it is possible to fill out an application and obtain an RN job, developing a resume will give you an edge over the competition. The most desired positions will have several to many people vying to be chosen, even during a nursing shortage. Your resume will make you stand out and help the recruiter, at a glance, identify you as an individual and a professional. A resume is your marketing tool. An updated resume will also help you keep stock of your certification/education deadlines and nursing-skill status.

There are several types of resumes. Usually, nurses use a chronological format (this is the style most recruiters prefer due to its ease of use), listing previous employers, the dates positions were held starting from the most recent and going backward. If you are a new graduate, this chronological format can be used to document key clinical experiences and educational milestones as well as your employment history.

A functional format resume can also be utilized if you don't have a lot of past work experience or have large gaps in employment (as a returning to the workforce RN might have). Functional resumes focus on categories of competency, such as technical skills, managerial ability, and those all-important (have we mentioned this lately?) transferable skills. Non-nursing employment experience can be utilized in this way but should be related to the skills important to the position you're seeking (e.g., sales gave you a unique perspective on quality public relations and service, etc.). A functional resume categorizes strengths and matches those strengths to the position you seek. Then, a job history is still listed, but in an abbreviated form and possibly on a second page.

If you can't decide which type to use, check out the box Functional or Chronological? If you're still unsure after that (and you have a fair amount of time on your hands) set up your information in both styles and then decide which one represents your skills and abilities most favorably. Regardless of the style you use, the key factors to any good resume are its accuracy, readability (clear, concise statements; attempt to limit the resume to one page), and inclusion of all necessary information.

Either way, here is a basic organizational format for a resume:

- Demographic information
- Education

Then,

- For chronological resumes—work experience, professional achievements, professional associations, relevant personal activities and awards, commendations, etc.

Functional or Chronological?

To help decide which resume format is best for you, ask yourself:

- Do I have a strong, consistent work history? This can be related to work in the field during nursing school.
- Is the position I'm applying for similar to my past work experience?

If so, use chronological format.
Otherwise, do you:

- Wish to highlight certain skills or abilities?
- Have gaps in your employment history?
- Have a history of changing jobs frequently?
- Need to focus strongly on transferable skills?

Then, use the functional format.

- For functional resumes—strength/skill categories (relating to desired skills of the position in question), professional/educational award and achievements, community activities (e.g., volunteer work, etc.) and connected honors, after which you finally list work experience.

The first section of a resume should contain demographics: name, address, telephone number, and e-mail address. Make sure the telephone number you're giving is connected to voicemail without a zany welcome message. You don't want your prospective employer to be greeted by "Hi, you've reached the loony bin," or belching sounds or the like.

The next category will list your educational history starting with degrees in progress and then the most recently achieved degree(s). Include the school's names and state in which it is located. For new graduates and for those using the functional format, mention any special awards and recognitions at this point. In the functional format it is also appropriate to discuss clinical experience and associated skill-building activities. Your grade point average can be included if you are a very new grad and you want to include it.

The rest of the order of your resume will depend on your chosen format. For work experience in a chronological resume, you will list your previous employers starting from the present time and going back. Document the employer's name, city, and state, your job title, dates of employment, and a brief profile of your responsibilities. Include any leadership situations or specialized skills. Organize the statement so that progression of your expertise and leadership responsibilities is reflected (e.g., in-services you conducted, mentorship, charge activities, etc.) at the end of the description. In addition, to highlight career and capability development, focus on the achievements in the most recent positions. For instance, use bulleted lists to highlight three key accomplishments per position and use action verbs: implemented, created, facilitated, increased, etc.

Again, it's appropriate to mention non-nursing positions, but lead the reader to see the connections between the skills obtained during your non-nursing employment that you will use during your nursing career, hopefully at their facility.

Under a separate heading list all licensures, certifications, etc. List all professional and educational association memberships. Use the full name of the organization, not their abbreviations.

For the personal activities segment, list community and volunteer activities, involvement with school/parent organizations, positions held in neighborhood organizations or in local government, etc. Mention any awards or commendations you have received. With these and all honors, cite the year you received it and the awarding organization.

This section can be quite helpful for providing insight into your personality and it will help a recruiter see you as an individual. It also can flesh out a resume that may be somewhat spare in other sections. The concept is to help the potential interviewer see you as a motivated desirable employee prospect. Things to avoid mentioning are marital status, race, age, religion, or sexual orientation. These factors are not relevant to choosing or not choosing an employee and should therefore be omitted. Also, in the spirit of keeping it short, sweet, and again relevant, it's not necessary to list leisure time hobbies such as painting, horseback riding, chainsaw juggling, etc.

The whole kit (as well as the caboodle) must then be presented as an original document (not photocopied) on good-quality, white or off-white paper (no lavender or happy face paper please) in a 12-point font. The envelope should match the paper, and the entire product should be word processed, read out loud to check for awkward word progression, checked by your mother and 6th grade English teacher, and, well, we think you get the point—make sure it's a clean, professional, error-free document.

Now we have one more important piece to this puzzle,

The Cover Letter

This introduction (a.k.a. "cover") letter should be no more than two or three paragraphs in length, single spaced. It should address the specific person you're sending the resume to. If the correct title and name of the recruiter, etc., is not available from an advertisement, call the appropriate office to obtain the information. Make sure the person's name is spelled correctly and his/her credentials are documented accurately. Attention to detail will convey professionalism and carry over to the overall impression developed by the reader.

Mistakes, which employers may feel reveal complacency, at the onset will also carry over and may make the recruiter eliminate you as a prospect before even reading further.

After a general greeting ("Dear Ms. Jones"), state the purpose of your letter, naming the title of the position you are interested in. State how you heard about the opportunity (e.g., the name, date and location of the ad., the referring RN, etc.) The next paragraph should briefly and creatively present your qualifications for the position you wish to apply for.

The final paragraph should express your hope that the recruiter will contact you at his or her earliest convenience. State a date that you will make contact for follow-up and to offer any further information that may be necessary.

Then don't forget to do it (follow-up, that is)! In a cover letter, you are allowed to utilize writing that's interesting or has more personal flair when writing about your motivation and credentials. This is a personal introduction and even nurse recruiters get tired of reading the same-old, same-old, over and over again. Shock value or overly cutesy statements, however, should be avoided for obvious reasons.

In our increasingly cyber-directed world, a paper resume may not (gasp!) be enough. For a few tips on creating an electronic resume or an employment home page, see Making the Most of Online Employment Resources and Creating an Employment Home Page.

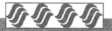

Making the Most of Online Employment Resources

The amount of job information available online can be overwhelming. To tame the wilds of the cyberspace job search jungle you have to know not only what you're looking for but also the best type of places to find it. Here are some tips to help you with your search:

1. Before you start any specific job searching net session, plan a bit. Write down exactly what you're looking for and how much time you plan to spend. It sounds anal-retentive, but if you're like one of us (Kelli) who loves to follow link after link after link after link you can easily start out researching travel nursing opportunities in Guam and soon find yourself reading an online comic book about the history of bubble gum.
2. If you've already investigated some fields of practice in Chapter 3, you may have a collection of bookmarks of places you've visited. You can revisit these sites now, with an eye toward obtaining a specific job rather than just searching for more general information.
3. There are different types of job search Websites (a number are listed in the Resources section of this chapter, along with the special features, benefits, and drawbacks of each of them), some more useful than others.

Probably the most comprehensive of the nursing job search sites are the nursing employment clearinghouses or nursing employment Websites created in conjunction with a regional print magazine. Think Nursing Spectrum (www.nursingspectrum.com) or Advance for Nurses (http://www.advancefor-nurses.com). The nice thing about these Websites is that they contain pages and pages of archived articles about many different aspects of nursing employment as well as classifieds ads, etc.

(continued)

Next in order of usefulness are the Web-only nursing or health care specific sites. Two of the largest are Nursezone.com and Hospitalsoup.com. These often have great search capabilities but not as many archived articles as Websites in the first category.

Finally, there are general employment search Websites, the biggest of which is monster.com. These sites can be potentially useful because they usually have some nursing jobs listed. However, on many general sites you have to search through listings for home health aids, nursing assistants, etc., which the keyword "nursing" or "nurse" brings up. Try searching with "RN" as the keyword instead.

When choosing which online job-search sites to use, consider such things as:

- Does the site help you format a resume (i.e., with a forms function) which the site then sends (at your request) to selected employers?
- Does the site allow you to post your resume anonymously? This may be useful if your current employer doesn't know you are looking for a job and you don't want them to know.
- Does the site provide e-mail addresses for job seekers? For example, www.employawonderfulnurse.com might provide registered users with NancyNurse@employawonderfulnurse.com. This can be useful so that you don't have to give out pookiepie@snippetysnip.com or whatever your home e-mail address is. This is a good idea from both a professional standpoint and to prevent spam from flooding your home box.
- Does the site provide a job tracking service? For example, some sites will allow you to set criteria for desired employment and will then e-mail you with the information when jobs meeting your criteria are posted. The more specifically you can set your criteria, the more helpful this feature will be for you. If you only want to see inpatient pediatric jobs paying more than $50,000 a year that are less than 2 miles from you in Perkasie, Pennsylvania, you are going to get fewer unhelpful job leads in your mailbox than if you can only set the parameters for inpatient care within a three-state area.

Practicing Your Employment Interviews

When all of your hard work pays off and you're scheduled for a job interview, rejoice! Then, practice and prepare! You will be much more at ease during an interview if you have worked through what you want to present about yourself and have thought about questions you and the interviewer may ask.

You will also need to be knowledgeable about the institution you'll be interviewing with. It is very important that you research the facility in the reference section of its library, via the Internet, career guides, nursing department, public relations department, etc. Collect a patient-care handbook if available. Get an employee handbook. Print (and bring with

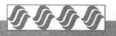

Creating an Employment Home Page

Does an RN applying for a staff nurse position need an employment home page?

Honestly? Probably not. Nevertheless, having a home page can be useful because you can post information on your page that won't fit on a resume. For example, a home page can showcase presentations you've developed, papers or articles you've written, and can provide more extensive details about your experience or skills.

Some tips for developing your home page:

- Although the days of free Web space are all but over, many Internet service providers include a small amount of server space for a site as part of the perks that come with the basic monthly fee.
- You don't need to have specialized computer skills to create a simple Web page. Even the monolithic, low-cost Web hosting companies provide page-building software that requires little more computer knowledge than knowing how to use a mouse. Homestead.com has a particularly user-friendly interface and avoids most of the "supercutsey" look of pages created through some of the other hosting companies.
- When designing your page, keep away from light-colored writing on a dark background because this can be extraordinarily difficult to read. Also, resist the urge to use animated cursors. While a blinking Band-Aid cursor is undeniably adorable, animated cursors are infamously buggy and occasionally even cause computer crashes.

you to the interview) a copy of the job description. Also via administration and/or the nursing department, you can obtain an organizational chart so you'll be familiar with the names of the CEO, CNO, COO, etc. Also collect a copy of the mission statement if available. This is where your informational interviewing data will again come in handy.

Invariably, an interviewer will ask you why you want to work at their establishment. If you know the employer's goals and ideology, you can give an intelligent answer to this.

Attempt to schedule the interview at a time of day when you are at your best. Find out the correct name and title of the persons you will be interviewed by and greet them by name when you meet them. Find out parking availability, if applicable. Make sure you know how to get to the interview (the good ol' trial run is still a good idea). In other words, the more prepared you are the calmer you will be. This will allow you to represent yourself at your most polished and professional. Often one candidate for a job is chosen over another because of how they present themselves, not solely because of their qualifications. This is especially true when applicants have similar levels of experience and expertise.

Don't forget to bring at least one copy of your resume to offer at the time of the interview Make sure you have included a list of five professional references, with name, phone number, and contact address for each (this should be presented on the same paper as your resume). If possible, you can obtain the facility's application and complete it ahead of time as well. All this will be duly noted by the recruiter and will have an impact on his or her decision.

We know you already know that when you go on the actual interview you have to be professionally dressed, but as career guide authors, we're required by state law to remind you once again.

A suit in a subdued shade, proper shoes (no stilettos, no boondockers), paired with a proper briefcase or formal satchel to carry all papers and documents is the prerequisite uniform. Do not try to impress (or knock out) the recruiter with your cologne and keep makeup very toned down. Also bring copies of all certifications, any thank you letters from patients, licenses, honors, etc., compiled in a neat folder that can be offered to the interviewer.

After you have compiled all of your data, you should take some time and write down questions. These will be questions you want to ask your prospective employer and questions you think the interviewer may ask you. Interviewers will ask you a few basic types of questions:

- Background questions for clarification of your resume. These could be related to previous work experience, school experience, etc.
- Professional questions about career goals, such as "What do you see yourself doing in 5 to 10 years?" The interviewer is attempting to see if your aspirations match the needs of her facility.
- Behavioral questions. These help the interviewer gain insight into your skills and abilities. They are "how would you" questions, such as "How would you deal with an irate family member or coworker?" etc.

Prepare 3X5 cards with as many mock interview questions as you can think of and prepare succinct answers to them. Use examples whenever possible to illustrate your point. Let's say, for example, that an interviewer asked you the question, "How would you deal with a fellow employee who you felt was acting in an unethical way?" This is an example of a behavioral question. Behavioral questions are used to ascertain the degree to which you have developed the specific personality characteristics the recruiter is looking for. The question posed above would be used to evaluate your assertiveness and ethics as well as see if your ethical framework is similar to the ethics of the institution.

When answering this type of question, knowledge you have gained about the institution will again come in handy. Many employers have ethics hotlines or other mechanisms in place to help employees handle ethical issues. You could cite your knowledge about these processes and then briefly reiterate a scenario that you experienced in your work, student, or even other life, and how you handled the issue. Attempt to portray yourself in the most positive and professional light possible. For other questions, use any highlighted or emphasized traits found in the advertisement for the position to clue into what the interviewer may be looking for. You can also write a few brief (read: under 2 minutes) success stories that will further illuminate your answers. Develop answers that illustrate that you are ethical, flexible, able to think on your feet, endowed with fine communication skills, a team player, in possession of leadership ability, in possession of professional and healthy boundaries, impervious to stress (or at least a master at handling it), able to multitask, prioritize, and think critically.

Then it's time for some (drum roll please) role-play. Have a friend question you using your cards. Practice answering until the words flow and you feel confident in your answers.

Finally you should prepare questions to ask the interviewer. These generally are concrete issues related to insurance, tuition reimbursement, nurse-to-patient ratios, policies on pulling or "floating" nurses (often what happens when the census is low or when a unit is short staffed), shift rotation, and charge practices (who will you be supervising; ancillary staff, RNs, LPNs, etc.) You might also ask, "How is maternity/family leave handled and who is eligible? What is the weekend holiday work policy?"

You should also make a point to ask what the institution's philosophy of nursing is. Be prepared to be asked about your personal philosophy of nursing as well.

It is very important that you convey confidence and calmness via your body language during the interview. Give the interviewer your full attention and good eye contact. Do not sit all tied up like a pretzel with you arms crossed, legs crossed (eyes crossed) because this gives the impression (however false it may be) of defensiveness and dishonesty. Sit slightly forward and use a strong but conversational tone. Do not rush to answer questions, especially difficult ones. It is perfectly acceptable to say, "Now let me think about that for a minute." This can convey how seriously you are taking the question and reinforces sincerity on your part. Practice your handshake with willing volunteers in advance as well.

After your interview, and within 24 hours, send a typed thank you note to the persons who interviewed you. Thank them for their time and attention, and reiterate your desire to work at Hospital XYZ and that you look forward to hearing from him or her. If you receive no response after 1 to 2 weeks, call. If you do not receive an offer you still have honed your skills for the next interview (interviews that you should be scheduling in lumps for momentum and motivation's sake). Remember, cliché warning—practice makes perfect.

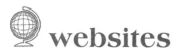 **websites**

Advance for Nurses
www.advancefornurses.com
An extremely useful nursing job search site. The site includes many ads for nursing openings that you can search by category or keyword. If you find a job opening that interests you, simply forward your resume to potential employers via e-mail or create a resume with the site's software. The site also has career resource links and loads of free articles about writing resumes and cover letters as well as all manner of job-search advice, articles about diversity in the nursing profession, patient handouts you can print and use, and helpful threaded discussion boards organized by topic. But wait, there's more. Advance also has separate listings and info for LPNs and lots of LPN job postings. You can also use their job messenger service and a handy-dandy "save this search for later" function.

Career Bookmarks at the Virtual Reference Library
http://careerbookmarks.tpl.toronto.on.ca/
This is a comprehensive site developed by the brilliant and industrious folks at the Toronto, Ontario, Public Library. Their strategy is to combine online information resources with links to paper resources (also known as books) for further info. Includes a step-by-step job search tutorial and sections on job search strategies, self assessment, career choices, marketing yourself, and success on the job.

The Damn Good Resume Site
www.damngood.com
This is the companion site to *The Damn Good Resume Book* by Yana Parker, a book which—according to the site—has the distinction of being the most frequently stolen resume book from libraries nationwide. This Web page is very approachable, with cute graphics and an easy-to-follow menu. It's particularly useful for someone needing the basics of resume writing and job interviewing. Starts with "What is a resume?" It has lots of tips and excellent questions and answers for different situations, such as adults entering workforce for the first time, adults in career transition, military folks transitioning to civilian work, and for young adults getting their first job. It includes quizzes to find talents/areas of strength that would be useful to review before an interview. Note that the site is filled with useful tips but is not a resume builder.

Discover Nursing
www.discovernursing.com/specialties.asp
This site includes a well-organized, comprehensive list of nursing specialty organizations, with links to each.

HTML Goodies
www.htmlgoodies.com
Thinking about building an employment home page but don't know where to start? Here would be a great place! This is a basic primer on building a Website for any reason; super nontechnical and friendly.

Job Hunt
www.job-hunt.org
Contains many interesting articles with information not found elsewhere, including our favorite, the "Dirty Dozen Online Job Search Mistakes." This site has a lot of information about, and emphasis on, protecting your privacy while job searching online. Don't forget to sign up for their free newsletter before you leave.

Job Yogi
www.jobyogi.com
This site contains many excellent articles about the nitty-gritty dynamics of job searching. For example, see their section on creating a scannable resume (includes information about how to use keywords) before you send out your resume to any medium- or large-sized company. Also includes information on salary negotiations and some interesting interview horror stories that will definitely make you feel better about your job search experience.

Nursing Spectrum
www.nursingspectrum.com
Another very comprehensive nursing job search site. In addition to a sizable collection of ads for open positions, this site also contains lots of free articles on resume writing, interviewing, etc. Don't miss the well-organized threaded discussion boards. Their job search is easy, chat rooms get some activity, and they have guest chats scheduled. Also check out their "Virtual Career Fair" for the ultimate in technology-meets-the-job-search experience.

Really Big
http://www.reallybig.com
Hey, guess why they call this site Really Big? Right, because it's really, really, really big. This site contains more than 5000 resources for Web

builders (that's you, when you're creating an employment home page) including free clipart, scripts, counters, fonts, html, java, animation, backgrounds, icons, buttons, photographs, etc., as well as information on site promotion and easy-to-follow Web-building tips.

Sigma Theta Tau List of Nursing Organizations

http://www.nursingsociety.org/career/nursing_orgs.html

This site also includes a list of nursing specialty organizations with links to each. Comprehensive and frequently updated.

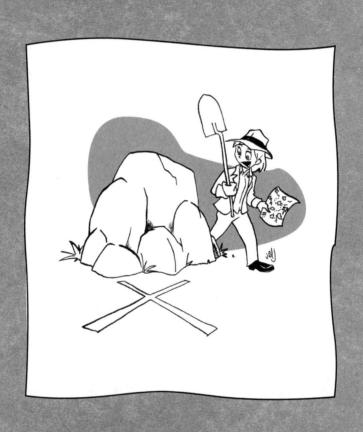

Looking for Jobs in All the Right Places

┌─ *A Nurse (Recruiter) Speaks* ──────────────────────

"If you've ever thought of moving to sunny Florida, now is the time. We have immediate openings for new grads at our magnet-status facility located just minutes away from Orlando theme parks and the white sands of Daytona Beach. We offer a $4000 sign-on bonus, relocation assistance, a supportive orientation and full tuition reimbursement for ongoing education. All shifts available, with weekends or holiday-free options. Free uniforms, free meals, assistance with housing and free trips to Disney World to meet personally with Mickey Mouse or your choice of beloved Disney characters. New grad positions are available in the CCU, ICU, NICU, L &D, OR and in the ED. Apply today at www.greatesthospitalintheworld.com and you can be on your way to our little bit of heaven tomorrow."

  —*Message from a nurse recruiter (only very slightly exaggerated) left on Kelli's answering machine while her area was being pounded by the worst snowstorm in 7 years.*

Can an Externship Become an Internship?

Perhaps the first place new grads look for work is right at the end of their stethoscope, in hospitals or other institutions where they have done a clinical rotation, or a unit they've worked on as a tech or extern. BL, who graduated 2 years ago, said, "I worked as a tech on the [OB] floor I'm on and wished to continue there as an RN.

Since I already worked there, I was offered the position, and I love my job."

The advantages for both the facility and the nurse in this scenario are numerous. First, both the facility and the new nurse are a known entity to the other. Especially if the nurse is going to be working on the same unit, he or she will not have to spend the first few weeks asking questions such as, "Um, what's the code to the clean linen room again?" or "How do I get to the computer screen that lets me order a replacement meal for a patient?" and can instead focus on adapting to the RN role. The nurse will also be familiar with the division of labor between the RNs/LPNs/techs as well as the intricacies of interunit politics. The facility saves money on recruiting a new nurse and doing another round of human resources paperwork (e.g., pre-employment physical, reference checks, etc.) and will most likely have a full-functioning RN sooner than if they had hired someone from outside who was unfamiliar with the unit.

There is a psychological advantage for the new grads also—knowing they have a job waiting, and knowing about the unit, the people who work there, and the patient population they typically serve can decrease feelings of insecurity and make the transition to RN a smoother one.

According to some new grads, however, the transition from CNA or tech to RN on the same unit can be about as smooth as sandpaper when other employees on the unit have difficulty accepting the RN's changed status. A new grad from California told us, "One day I was shooting the breeze with the other PCAs [patient care associates] and the next day they didn't want to have anything to do with me. I was in the position of having to direct them now that I was 'the nurse' and they didn't like it. Eventually, I just said 'you know, I'm sorry things are different now, but I'm the same guy I used to be. Do I have like bubonic plague all of a sudden? Why are you all avoiding me?' Ultimately, I think they knew I was going to be fair since I had been where they were, but the transition was really rough. I had to re-earn their trust." Other nurses, too, may have trouble seeing the new RN as a "real nurse," and it may take some time to shake off their image of you as either a tech or (as one new grad put it) "a bumbling, extremely wet behind the ears, tentative GN."

Ways RNs suggested to help mitigate difficulties with a change from tech to an RN status include: talking openly about the upcoming change with your fellow techs and nurses, reading up on the art of delegation (see the Resources section in Chapter 8) and role-playing delegation scenarios with fellow new grads or your nurse manager. In addition, a transfer to another unit in the same facility can provide some of the advantages of staying put at the same facility while giving the new grad the freedom to flourish in a new role.

Using Online Job Search Resources

So how can the Web help you find job openings? Well, to start with, there are the so-called super-portals, or generalized job search sites. A number of these sites are listed in the Resources section of this chapter, but the best site is monster.com, which has 24.5 million resumes posted. While these sites include "help wanted" listings for everything from aardvark trainers to xylophone repair technicians, most also contain plenty of listings of RN openings. Despite their massive size, finding nursing jobs through these sites is not impossible because most integrate highly specialized search capabilities (you can search using multiple key words, by region, by specialty, etc.) and the ability to post a resume so that employers come looking for you. Some sites have an option that allows you to post a resume anonymously (especially good if you don't want your current employer to know you're scouting around for another job) and some will keep track of new jobs that are posted each day that meet the parameters you've established.

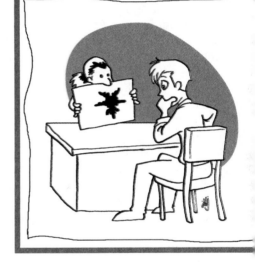

Most of the general sites don't differentiate between a position as a licensed nurse and what they call a "nursing" job (usually openings for certified nursing assistants). To avoid searching through trillions of CNA ads, use the search term "RN" or "LPN" instead of "nurse" or "nursing."

These generalized portals can be tremendously helpful, and many offer not only listings of job openings, but articles on subjects such as preparing a resume, tracking employment trends, what to wear to a job interview, how to negotiate and evaluate salary offers, etc. Many also contain extensive message boards to network with other job applicants and folks working in the field, which could come in particularly handy if you haven't yet been able to develop that new grad support group we keep bugging you about!

A few words of caution, however, these larger sites have recently started to issue warnings about fake job postings and identity theft, and caution job applicants to avoid giving out their social security number until they have researched their potential new employer through other means. With nursing jobs, this should be easy enough because information on most health-care facilities is available on the Web or through the appropriate accreditation/licensing body. See the Resources section of this chapter for pertinent Websites.

In addition to the general employment portals, there are many nursing-specific employment sites that can make the search easier for you. A few of the best are listed in the Resource section of this chapter, but be sure to access the updates for this book at the publishers' Website (www.fadavis.com) because these sites have been known to merge, change hands, or expand almost overnight. These sites also include informative articles, message boards, and chats, all targeted toward the job-searching nurse. Because these sites are nursing specific, this saves you wading through multiple pages about such compelling topics as the salary differences between a graduate of the Wharton MBA program and the Harvard MBA program, and allows you to more quickly access topics of real interest to you.

In general the use of these sites is free to the job hunter. Even listings that are placed by search companies (more commonly known as "headhunters") should ultimately charge the folks looking to hire, not you, for hooking you up.

Also, most larger newspapers now post their classified ads section online. Although perusing the classifieds online doesn't have the same feel as intently hunching over the newspaper "help wanted" section in a coffee shop (you know, like in the movies), it does make it easier to search for a specific job opening. Not only that, barring any strange problems with your keyboard or mouse, if you search online, you'll save yourself from having newsprint-smudged hands.

On the Web, you can also locate job openings in individual facilities as many larger facilities now carry job postings through their home page. Some even include a link to e-mail a resume or have an online form to request more information. While you're hanging out at a facility's Website, don't limit yourself to only looking around the human resources section. You can peruse the rest of the site and get a general flavor of what the facility is all about and what it would be like to work there (or at least what the public relations people would like you to think!). If you decide to apply, be sure to check out the facility's mission statement. It will give you valuable information about what the facility thinks is important, and if you ask a question about the mission statement in your interview, we can almost guarantee the nurse recruiter is going to be impressed.

The Web can also be used to do additional research on the facilities that most interest you. Do a news search (go to yahoo.com, click on news and continue with your search) to see what kind of press the facility has been getting. This is an excellent way to garner information about a facility not in your geographical area that the facility typically wouldn't include on its home page. A good example of such information is the presence of labor disputes. This can save inconveniences such as moving 2000 miles across the country to take a job at the "perfect" facility only to find out you have walked into a strike situation, that the hospital is located within the walls of a nudist colony, or that the Orlando hospital that sounded like a tropical dream come true pays staff only in Disney dollars.

Even if you are going to stick with the old standbys of using the newspaper and making phone calls for your job search, it's wise to provide an e-mail address on your resume, even if the facility may never use it. There are several reasons for this. First, it gives the impression that you are computer literate and up-to-date. This can be a concern for some returning nurses who may have a bit of gray around the temples. It's not legal for facilities to discriminate against you because you are older, but that doesn't mean it doesn't happen, and while it's a small step, it's simple enough to arm yourself with an e-mail address. You don't even need to have Internet access at home; just use one of the free Web-mail services (a sample of some that are available are listed in the Resources section of this chapter) and check your e-mail from the local public library.

In addition, as a busy new grad, you may be hard to reach, so e-mail correspondence may be more efficient, particularly if you are still working at your previous job. It's common sense and—to a lesser extent—common courtesy not to use the e-mail provided by your current employer to correspond with a potential new employer. Use the Web-based services instead, some of which even include the free use of an e-mail-to-fax number.

Finding Jobs Through the Classifieds

Of the many new grads and long-time nurses with whom we talked for this book, only a small fraction had ever taken a job they'd found through classified ads in their local paper. Most nurses had at least looked through the classifieds when engaged in a job search, but usually stated that they found that such a small percentage of nursing jobs were advertised in general newspapers that they had greater success through network referrals or ads found in the regional nursing employment periodicals.

So while the general classifieds are not necessarily the most useful tools for the nurse on a job hunt, it doesn't cost anything to look (okay, only 35 to 60 cents or so). In addition to alerting you to potential job openings, the classifieds can be a valuable source of information. By perusing them you can figure out what facilities are most desperate (look for sign-on bonuses in the four digits), what types of units certain facilities maintain (i.e., if they have multiple openings), and what kind of carrots (shift differentials, continuing education, your weight in chocolate) facilities are offering to persuade nurses to sign on.

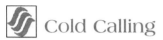 Cold Calling

No, it's not what happens when you use your cell phone from a street corner in Alaska in January. Cold calling is contacting a facility about a job even though you've seen no advertised position. You may be asking, "Why exactly would I call anyone when—because of the nursing short-age—nurse recruiters call me every day, offering trips, cash, an advanced degree, even a kidney if I will come to work at their hospital?"

This is a good question, astute reader, and the answer is quite simple—if you investigate job leads only from facilities that contact you, you are limiting your employment possibilities to working only at the facilities that are most desperate for nurses. There are many reasons a facility might be aggressively recruiting for nurses, even positive ones (e.g., the facility is adding a new unit or hiring additional nurses in order to decrease the patient-to-nurse ratio), but you may or may not know the real reasons until you are hired and on the floor. In the meantime, you might miss an excellent job that would be a better fit for you.

Another reason for cold-calling is that sometimes a job that might be filled quite nicely by a nurse isn't advertised as a nursing job. For exam-ple, being a case manager at a shelter for homeless people with mental illness might be a great fit for a nurse who has a specific skill set or expe-rience. However, the facility might not have thought of this possibility, or might prefer to advertise it to folks with a bachelor's degree in social work. Although these types of jobs are definitely not going to pay as well as a hospital job, if you're looking for a specific experience instead of a specific salary range, it may well work for you. Because jobs in the nonprofit sector are so infrequently advertised through venues such as the general classifieds, if you want a job in the nonprofit sector, the cold call will become your good friend. There are, however, some organiza-tions and Websites that help match potential employers with potential employees in the nonprofit world. Some of these are included in the Resources section of this chapter.

So if you know you would really like to work at your local children's hospital, or that you want to be the occupational nurse at the zoo, don't be afraid to contact them even if you don't see an ad. Most larger facilities have Websites where you can find relevant contact information, including the postal and e-mail address of their human resources department. When making a first time contact via e-mail, don't include your resume as an attachment, or it may well be deleted by a virus-wary personnel assistant. Call or e-mail first to see if it's okay to send an attachment, and then you can put "requested resume" in the subject line. Alternatively, you can post your resume on your Website and send the URL.

 ## Making the Most of Network Referrals

Although the word networking has unfortunately taken quite a beating (one nurse we talked with said, "Ah, yes, networking, in other words, manipulating human contact for the purposes of personal gain."), it's a buzzword that has stubbornly refused to fade away. This is probably because the real concept behind it is a good and necessary one; chat rooms and virtual reality notwithstanding, human contacts pave the way for human achievement.

At any rate, we prefer the term "community-building" to "networking" because we feel it more closely describes what nurses need to do to develop a professional support circle.

You've already done plenty of community-building. You probably have at least a few instructors, classmates, and hospital personnel with whom you worked in clinical rotations who would be glad to give you hand with your professional development, including letting you know of any job possibilities that might be brought to their attention.

Since we know you already started the new grad support group we mentioned in the first chapter of this book, hopefully all your fellow job seekers are keeping their eyes out for employment possibilities that might be a good match for you, as you are for them.

If you didn't ask any instructors if you could use them as referrals, now is the time to send a chatty e-mail (you can find their e-mail, if needed, through the search function on your school's Website) and ask. This will not only secure a potential reference provider for you, but will also give the instructor an opportunity to pass along a job possibility he or she might have heard of that would match what you're looking for. Clinical faculty who are adjunct and full-time at the hospitals might be in a special position to recommend you to their friendly neighborhood nurse recruiter or let you know the inside scoop on whether working on a particular unit would be the greatest thing since sliced bread or the worst idea since fried Spam.

Acing the Interview: Know Your Nurse Recruiter

Most interviewing advice is stuff you already know to do—arrive on time, dress appropriately, don't chew gum, listen to the interviewer, watch your body language, offer a firm (not bone-crunching) handshake, make eye contact, smile.

All the same, this book just wouldn't be considered a real career guide if we didn't include a few words about how to make a favorable in-person impression.

It's not essential, but it makes life easier for you if you have a conservative blue suit so you never have to worry about finding something perfectly appropriate to wear to an interview. And as for other appearance issues, remember you want the interviewer to be struck by your awe-inspiring intelligence, plentiful people skills, and colossal amount of clinical knowledge. If he or she is at all distracted by your appearance, that's what the interviewer will be thinking about. Not fair, but true. Many handbooks for the job seeker suggest covering up piercings and tattoos. Having a pierced septum or a Bugs Bunny tattoo on your wrist could not possibly be more unrelated to your ability to provide good nursing care. Nevertheless, a tattoo or a piercing might distract the person interviewing you, so for now, it may make your life easier if you temporarily take it out or cover it up. If it pains you to put on the suit and take out the piercing, think of yourself as dressing up for a play in which you and the job interviewer have the lead. You'll be able to take off the costume soon enough. The nursing profession needs folks with a strong sense of individuality, but no matter how bad the nursing shortage gets, you probably won't get the job if you show up for the interview in combat boots and a bathing suit.

To go with your blue suit, it's great to have a hard-sided portfolio case instead of a backpack. The portfolio will keep your papers neater and in better order than a backpack, but is cheaper (not to mention less ostentatious) than a briefcase.

If you're not familiar with the facility where you will be interviewing, it's a good idea do a dry run to the facility before the day of your interview. This way you'll know your directions are good, that you can find parking if needed, etc. If possible, locate a coffee shop (preferable to a diner, to prevent walking into the interview accompanied by the smell of fried breakfast food clinging to your clothes) where you can wait if the transportation gods are with you and you arrive extra early on the day of the interview.

In addition to your spiffy portfolio, make sure you take the following to an interview: extra copies of your resume, an extra pen, copies of your license and diploma and possibly child abuse/police checks, which are required in some community health arenas. Also have a word-processed list of three to five references and their contact info. Some nursing job search gurus advise having business cards with your name and address printed up, but most nurses we talked with thought that might be a little overkill when applying for a staff nurse position.

As for the mechanics of the interview, the most important part of being able to answer a question is to listen carefully to the question itself. You can also repeat the question back to the interviewer to show you are listening as well as give yourself time to formulate the answer. If it's a tricky question, or if you don't quite understand what the interviewer is asking, ask him or her to rephrase it. The interviewer has been undoubtedly asking the same things all day, and may forget that it's a new question to you.

Since you've probably interviewed for a job or two in your lifetime, this process is not a new one, although you may be surprised by your level of anxiety surrounding an interview. This is normal; you're starting a new profession. You may have interviewed for a job as a banker, or baker, or even a candlestick maker, but this is a new role so it feels different.

A word of encouragement, even your annoying classmate who thinks she's Florence Nightingale reincarnated and knew she wanted to be a nurse since she was 7-days-old still doesn't feel like a real nurse yet. Here's where the age-old adage (or is it a new-age catch-phrase) "fake it till ya make it" comes in. You graduated from nursing school, right? You passed (or will pass) the NCLEX, right? Well, then, you're a nurse. You may be an inexperienced nurse, but you're a nurse, and your profession needs you.

The interviewer probably isn't out to stump you, just figure out what kind of employee you will be, so the chances are good that most questions asked are going to be the standard interview fare you've heard many times before. And even if the questions are very nursing-specific or even very unusual (e.g., "If you were an extinct animal what kind of extinct animal would you be?"), take a deep breath and give it your best shot. Remember, you've had experience thinking on your feet every day in clinical. When Mr. Brown in Bed 27A asked, "Aren't you too young/old/male/to be a nurse?", or the 7-year-old during your pediatric rotation wanted to know, "Do kids ever die when they get their tonsils out?", you came up with an answer, didn't you?

You can rehearse virtual interviews with an interactive computer program that asks you questions and responds to your response. These are available online through sites like monster.com. There are some limitations. It is a computer program, and a general one, so it won't ask your nursing-specific questions, but it can be a good starting place for practice, particularly if you haven't interviewed in a while or haven't had an actual professional level interview. You can also buy or borrow a job interview question book (some of the better ones are listed in the Resources section of this chapter) and practice interviewing with your new grad support group, spouse, or children or even a particularly articulate family pet. When practicing, don't forget to prepare answers to some behavioral-type questions. More information on answering this type of question can be found in the box Answering Behavioral Questions.

It's important to have some questions of your own, including perhaps some that you will develop by considering your most important job criteria through the process described in Chapter 4. The more specific questions you can ask about the facility (e.g., "I read on your Website that this hospital places a great deal of emphasis on the RN as a 'lifetime learner.' What kind of continuing education do you offer?"), the more relevant information you will obtain. You will also show you have prepared for the interview. Especially if the nurse recruiter has had a long day (and probably has), the recruiter will appreciate the effort you've put into your preparation.

Finally, to deal with anxiety, realize that you do have choices. When one of us (Kelli) was finishing her AD, an instructor asked a nurse recruiter from a local facility (we'll call it "Hospital X") to present some tips about acing a nursing interview. The tip Kelli remembered most vividly was the nurse recruiter's insistence that skirts, heels, earrings and full make-up were essential for all female interviewees. Like many nurses, Kelli is really not a make-up and heels kind of gal. At that point, she was willing to do the blue suit, but couldn't imagine working someplace that seemed so interested in enforcing stereotypical female appearance norms. All Kelli wrote in her class notebook that day was "reminder to self: don't apply at Hospital X."

Kelli now works as a nurse home visitor in an area of Philadelphia where more casual dress is not just accepted, but essential.

The point is that unless your next month's rent will have to come from the local loan shark or you live in an isolated area where it's either

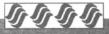

Answering Behavioral Questions

When interviewers use behavioral questions, they are looking for a situation in which interviewees demonstrated particular characteristics or for evidence that they have developed or used a skill the employer is looking for.

A typical behavioral interview question might be: "Can you tell me about a job experience in which you had to speak out against a situation that you thought was unjust?" In this case, the interviewer is trying to ascertain if the applicant is ethical and assertive.

Your answers to this type of question should be concrete, succinct, and detailed. They should portray you in the best possible light. As much as you'll be tempted to break the tension, now is not the time to bring out the humorous stories about your childhood experiences in summer camp. Ideally, use anecdotes from your clinical rotations or past work experience. For example:
Interviewer: Tell me about a time when you used creative problem-solving skills.
Good answer: During my community health rotation, I made a medication instruction chart with pictures on it for a patient who had difficulty reading.
Not as good: Before I had a remote control for my TV, I connected a string to the control knob so I could change channels without getting up from my chair.

One exercise you can do to prepare for behavioral questions in a job interview is to jot down a scenario or two that can be used to illustrate traits an employer might be looking for. If the job you are interviewing for is advertised, you can get ideas from the ad (for example, if the words "flexibility a must" are printed in bold). You can also get ideas from the following list:

What have you done that illustrates that you are:

- Ethical
- Flexible, able to think on your feet
- Articulate
- Endowed with good communication skills (written and spoken)
- Willing to go "above and beyond" the call of regular job responsibilities
- Able to maintain flexible but effective boundaries
- Able to deal with stress
- Able to juggle multiple tasks and prioritize
- Able to work on a team
- Able to think critically

Source: Adapted from Dunham, K: How to Survive and Maybe Even Love Nursing School. ed 2. F.A. Davis, Philadelphia, 2004, p 216, with permission.

working in the local community hospital or tending llamas, relax! You do have choices.

 ## After the Interview

After the interview, do some Monday morning quarterbacking. What went well in the interview? What did you wish you had done differently? Did any questions stump you? If you talked about salary in the interview, were you comfortable in the negotiations? Is there anything you could do to become more comfortable? If you took a tour, did you gain any information that might help you make a decision about whether this is the facility for you?

Finally—and pardon us while we channel your mother—don't forget to write a thank-you note for the interview. It can take less than 5 minutes if you have the supplies with your job hunting kit, and it's a relatively painless way to remind the nurse recruiter of your existence. It's also just a kind and polite (and somewhat expected) thing to do.

If you can add any sincere praise for something positive in the interview process, it wouldn't hurt to do so. Nurse recruiters have a hard job these days, and taking an extra moment to show appreciation is a nice gesture.

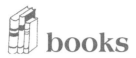 books

Adams, Bob (2001).
The Everything Job Interview Book. Avon, MA: Adams Media.

Truly does include everything, with an eye to helping the interviewee feel confident (see? Who needs the word "dummies" in the title). Includes information about various interview formats, including computer assisted interviews, as well as tons of examples of interview questions you might be asked. The handiest part of this guide is that it breaks up questions into groups based on what the interviewee is trying to discern, e.g., your ability, compatibility with company goals, your driving forces, special situations, etc.

Darke, John (1997).
The Perfect Interview: How to Get the Job You Really Want.
New York, NY: American Management Association.

This is the most comprehensive book on interviewing we came across in research for this chapter. It includes information on everything from the science behind networking calls to the many different kind of interviews, and interview questions (including questions you should avoid asking) as well as numerous worksheets to help you through preparing for the interview.

Dixson, Pam (2000).
Job Searching Online for Dummies. Hoboken, NJ: IDG Books.

Although we don't particularly like the idea of buying any book that advertises that it's for "dummies," we still recommend this one. One of the book's best features is the inclusion of a free CDROM that links to relevant sites and other material. This book is not specific to nursing but contains valuable explanations of resume formatting for the Web, and information about developing an employment home page as well as detailed reviews of all the major general employment sites.

Fry, Ron (2000).
101 Great Answers to the Toughest Interview Questions.
Franklin Lake, NJ: Career Press.

This is another very good interview book and is an especially good bargain if you already know how to dress, make phone calls, follow-up, etc., and just need access to some practice questions. It's also light-hearted and might make you laugh out loud in a few places, which is somewhat rare in the career search guide genre (current book excepted of course). Also available on CD.

Resources

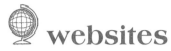 **websites**

Campus RN
www.campusrn.com
This site, designed for nursing students and entry-level heath-care students, contains a job search area, a resume builder, the potential to post resumes, and an area to research more than 50 hospitals in their database. This site also has a question and answer area that allows students to send in questions to be answered online. The site offers cash referral bonuses to registered members who refer other members to the site as well as loan consolidation advice. Perhaps the most compelling reason to register at this site is the scholarship center. Each year this site bestows six $2,500 scholarships to members currently enrolled in baccalaureate or graduate level programs with a 3.25 GPA or above. You go, campusrn.com!

Cool Works
www.coolworks.com
Fluorescent lights got you down? Cruise on over to this cool site chock full of outdoor jobs. You can't search by job title, instead the site lists the jobs in categories such as camp jobs, national park jobs, ski resort jobs, etc. If you don't find a nursing job here at first, keep checking back for new listings. Or take a summer off and be a camp counselor!

Hospital Soup
www.hospitalsoup.com
Don't let the goofy name fool you, this is a serious health-care–related job search site. Here you can access a job search, use e-mail notification, read career profiles, search international jobs, and sign up for a job search newsletter. You can also download patient information educational material here. The job search area only worked with specific words, i.e., worked with "RN" but not with "nursing." However, the Health/Medical library had tons of articles and video topics.

Job Search.org
www.jobsearch.org
This site is easy to use with up to 47 pages of nursing jobs listed at a time. Although the postings are current, there are non-RN jobs that come up in the search. The site allows online applications and you can post a resume and cover letter to a particular employer, to a few selected job postings, or online for all potential employers to see. The site also has a resume builder and tips on job hunting, interviewing, and salary negotiation. The site doesn't require a login but one is available, which allows job searches to be saved and you can register to create an auto job search that will e-mail you new postings.

Med Search
www.medsearch.com

WOW! This is the most comprehensive site we visited. Owned and operated by Monster, this site includes a job search function, resume builders, a career advice center, and even workplace tips. The job search section is easy to use and nets basically the same results as a general Monster search but is tailored to specific health-care fields, so a nursing search results in nursing jobs. Searches can be refined to location, company, and specialty. The resume center includes a resume builder, tips and samples, all tailored by specific industry, and the ability to post the resume online. The advice center offers tips on salary info, discussion boards, relocating advice, and specific areas about diversity. Make sure to check out the health-care features that include more than 30 articles on topics such as mandatory overtime, how to make it through the night shift, and how to handle difficult patients. There are also resources for people interested in volunteer opportunities domestic and international. It's a lovely all-purpose occupational resource.

Nursezone
www.nursezone.com

Nursezone is a comprehensive nursing Website and includes much more than the average job search site. Pages include a job search site, news articles sorted by specialty, a student nurse center, travel nursing resources, and relocation tools. The job search site results in general openings for travel positions in the specialty and geographic area of the user's choosing. The student nurse center includes resources on school selection, financial assistance, study tips and tools, and NCLEX prep. The site also offers ecards and pages of articles on relationships and caring for yourself.

Saludos
www.saludos.com

Job search site for Hispanic/Latino workers with a link to a health-care job search that allows nurses to browse through lists by specialty. There is a place to post resumes and an area for employers specifically looking for bilingual employees. There is a login required that can be used anonymously and is free. However, you do have to post a resume in order to search the jobs bank.

Yahoo Hot Jobs
hotjobs.yahoo.com

You can search for jobs by geographic area, title, function, and keywords here. Typical Yahoo style—easy on the graphics, easy on the eyes, quick to download.

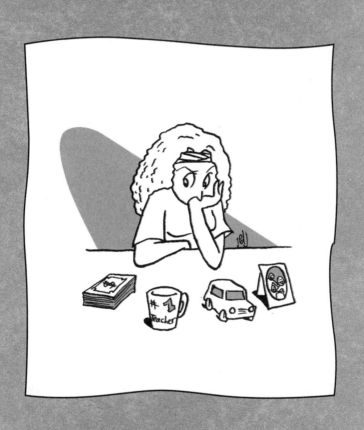

What's in It for Me: Considering Opportunities

A Nurse Speaks

"The salary was not [what made me decide my current job was right for me]. There are a lot of higher paying positions I could have taken. The location is great, it's a 15 minute drive. I had worked there for a while as a tech so knew the people I'd be working with and I liked them. I also knew what I'd be getting into when I took the job. Basically, I love what I do. If I were looking for benefits or pay I'd find another job."

BL, RN, Newborn nursery grad 2002

You are fully in the thick of the job search jungle now. You've located some potential employers, done your research, and had a few interviews. In Chapter 1, we talked about making an initial assessment of what you want in a job (perhaps your number-one priority), but now that you have lots more information (and undoubtedly some actual job offers) it's time for real decision making.

You have to make one big decision (which job to take), but it may be helpful to think of it as a series of smaller decisions about your priorities. For example, is it important to you to work at a teaching institution? Do your outside commitments (e.g., family) necessitate that you work a certain shift? Do you want to be within walking/cycling distance of your job? Do you need immediate cash to pay back Oscar, your friendly neighborhood loan shark? In this chapter, we'll examine some of the many different factors nurses weigh when considering job offers.

Institutional Variations

Of course, the first institutional variation question is, do you want to work in an institution? This book draws heavily from the experience of hospital nurses, since hospitals are the biggest employers of nurses. However, we would be remiss if we didn't mention there are tons of jobs nurses can do outside the hospital, from patient care coordinator at a primary care clinic to staff nurse on a movie set (providing first aid to Brad Pitt might be one nurse's dream and another nurse's nightmare!). Regardless of the type of facility or job you are considering, some of the questions below may be ones for you to consider:

How important to you is the issue of working in a nonprofit versus for-profit facility? Almost all of the nurses we talked with for this book reported that their facilities were actively engaged in cost-cutting measures, whether they were for-profit or not. The difference, nurses noted, is really about why these cost-containment measures are in place. "I work for a nonprofit community hospital in a rural area," said one 22-year veteran, "and we recently went to a really crummy benefit system to save money. If I worked for one of those monolithic for-profit hospital chains I would have been furious. I'm not saying I like it, but I know [the administration] is cutting costs so we can stay open. We're the only hospital for, literally, miles. The whole community comes here for care. I don't want it on my conscience that my next door neighbor died of an MI on the way to a distant hospital because I didn't want to pay a ten-dollar co-pay for my prescriptions."

Do you want to work at a teaching facility? Most nurses we spoke with agreed that there are many positive aspects to working in a teaching facility. For example, the attending docs in a teaching facility are almost always going to be up to date with the latest information and research, which makes it easier for the nurse to be as well. In addition, many nurses said they felt good about working in a teaching facility because they believe patients benefit from the extra time and attention a teaching facility afforded the patients, although it sometimes means patients have to "tell their story" a number of times.

In addition, some of the nurses who work in teaching hospitals said that knowing there were students/learners of all types around helps them be especially mindful of the care they give. One traveling nurse said, "When I am rotating through a teaching hospital, I always feel—how does that song go '…like somebody's watching me.' It's true. There are always eyes on you, observing, watching how you do things. I try harder to do them the right way, instead of the almost right way."

Of course, all these "eyes" hanging out means nurses do plenty of teaching, too. You will be a part of the process of educating students/interns/residents about everything from where the bathroom is to how to start an IV. Some nurses find this invigorating (or at least fun) while other nurses quickly become weary with the whole scene. Nurses also noted that in a teaching facility many processes (especially the admission process) can be longer because more people have to have their hands in it.

Is it important to you to work in a hospital with a nurses' union? Although being a part of a union doesn't guarantee anything approaching blissful working conditions (particularly if the union is weak and/or has ineffective leadership), the union will give the individual nurse (theoretically at least) backing in disputes, disagreements about appropriate nurse-to-patient ratios, and backing at contract negotiation time. Ideally, through collective bargaining, unionized nurses can ensure that the concerns of nurses and not just the concern of the shareholders or the bottom line are taken

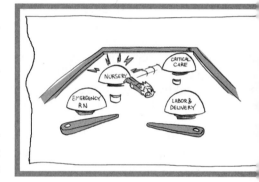

into account when administrative decisions are made. Unions sometimes provide additional benefits such as assistance with educational costs or direct training. In addition, many nurses involved in a union report that it helps them feel—pardon the cliché here—empowered. Their thoughts were similar to those of Sara Wendroff, who has been working as an RN in California for 15 years, " It's a shame nurses have to unionize, but we do. Nurses are extremely important to the health care system but we're just now demanding that level of professional power. Unions are an important part of our standing up for ourselves as professionals."

Do you want to work in a level one trauma center? Working at a level one trauma center practically guarantees that you will see patients with certain types of injuries, including those from gunshot wounds, severe motor vehicle accidents, stabbings, assaults, and rape. Even at the less acute stage, these type of injuries can be particularly challenging to your nursing skills, and can be extremely draining emotionally as well. Many nurses thrive on this challenge. As one nurse said, "They call me 'Exit Wound Ed' around the ED because I'm great at figuring out where the bullet came out, a lot better than even the docs that have been around a long time. I have to admit, I get an adrenaline rush when I hear "GSW" on our radio and we know someone is on their way."

Awaiting a gun shot victim might sound like Dante's fifth circle of hell to many nurses, for "Exit Wound Ed" it was a welcome challenge. If you find yourself relating to Exit Wound Ed, a level one trauma center might well be your proverbial cup-o-tea, although you needn't be as enthusiastic as Ed to consider the possibility. This is definitely one of those cases where "nurse, know thyself" is especially relevant advice.

Do you want to work for just one facility or would agency work better meet your needs? For the new grad, agency work can be extremely tough but with a good orientation and the right support it's certainly possible. The advantage of agency work is that there is usually a lot of flexibility and a higher rate of pay, although most often with decreased (or no) benefits. Another one of the advantages of working for an agency is that it can be very intensive experientially; you get to see many different types of patients and facilities in a short time. Of course, for a new nurse struggling to get oriented in a new profession, having to be oriented at a new facility every week might be an additional (and unwanted) challenge.

If you are thinking about agency nursing, you may want to consider how important it is for you to feel part of a team. The temporary nature of agency assignments (even long-term assignments, which hospitals try to avoid because of the cost) may mean you will not have the "team" experience and you may also miss out on the long-term friendships that often develop in the workplace.

Another question to consider is, *do you want to work in a small town, urban area, rural area, or something in between?* Of course, this may be a ready-made decision for you, based on where you live and how willing you are to commute. If you own a home in the isolated area surrounding Podamaquassy, Nebraska, aren't interested in moving, and don't want a long commute, then congrats ... Podamaquassy Community Hospital probably has just the nursing position for you.

However, if your situation is such that you can be a bit more flexible, you may want to consider some geographical factors when investigating jobs.

Some nurses find that they enjoy the diversity of the patient (and staff!) populations and more intense nature of the work in an urban hospital. Others like the intimate feel of their small town's own community hospital. We were interested to find, however, that many nurses who like community hospital nursing don't like to do it in their own town. "If my next door neighbor had a mastectomy, I only want to know because she wants to share with me, not because I've emptied her Foley bag post-op," explained a nurse from rural Wyoming, who finds that it's worth her 60-mile round trip commute to a hospital in a neighboring town where the patients are not all her neighbors.

Of course, this brings us to the topic of the commute and how long is too long, which is, of course, a matter not only of personal preference but also energy level. If you consider your commute part of your work day and you are going to be doing 12-hour shifts, a 45 minute commute means each working day will be no less than 14 hours. The costs of this, physically and emotionally, are going to be pretty substantial, especially if you are a recent grad suffering from those low-down-I-have-so-much-to-learn-that-they-didn't-teach-me-in-nursing-school blues, a.k.a. "new profession exhaustion." Craig Sanders, a PICU nurse from New York state cautioned, "Don't think that just because you commuted 2 hours a day in your pre–nursing school days that you will be happy with that kind of commute with a nursing job. Especially your first year out, take it easy on yourself, work as close as possible to your home."

If you choose to (or have to) commute, there are a number of ways you can make your commuting time more productive or at least more pleasant. This may involve listening to books on CD while driving, consciously using the time to decompress from your day, or as Staci sometimes does, picking a more picturesque driving route, even if it takes you a little out of your way.

Also, even if you have a car, look into your public transit options. Depending on the parking at your workplace, schedules, traffic, and availability of employer-provided assistance with public transportation costs, public transit may actually be cheaper and more convenient than driving. In addition, if you're taking public transit you can read, start on the historical young adult novel you've always wanted to write, and even catch a few zzz's, although probably not all at the same time.

Earning While You Learn: Preceptorship and Orientation Parameters

"A good orientation is every bit as much of a benefit as a great health insurance plan or a generous sign-on bonus," said Lyle Preston, who graduated from nursing school 2 years ago and is working in the NICU of a large urban hospital in Texas, "except for, as a new grad, I think a good orientation is more essential."

Most of the nurses we talked with agreed that not only is a good orientation program and a reliable, competent, preceptor important from a practical standpoint, but also from a symbolic one. "If hospitals care about nurses—and if they care about patients—they will take the time and trouble to design an orientation period and program that works," said RT, a 17-year veteran, "even as I've gotten farther along in my career and changed jobs, I've always chosen to work places that do a lot more than throw a couple of manuals at you and say 'holler if you have any questions.' "

What then, does a "good" orientation consist of? The answer to this question, like many in this book, is "it depends." An orientation should—in the words of one nurse—"keep you from feeling like you are being fed to sharks." Or at least, we might add, keep you from feeling like you're being fed to the sharks your very first day.

For new grads and nurses transitioning to a more complex or new area of practice, in order to not feel like shark food, they might need an orientation period that includes classroom training and instruction for needed certifications, and a series of clinical experiences with a preceptor and the new nurse working together, with the new nurse taking more and more responsibility as time goes on. In addition, many institutions include a series of return demonstrations or hands-on testing in needed hospital-based and unit-based competencies, and ask both experienced and new nurses to complete them. Orientation periods usually last from 4 to 12 weeks.

For the new grad taking a job where they have worked, for example, as a patient care tech the entire time they were in school, this may seem excessive, but many new grads told us the extensive process increased their confidence in themselves and their new role, and as an added bonus, increased their coworkers' confidence in them. "When my little initials on my name tag went from CNA to GN to RN I was afraid that people would never stop seeing me as 'the tech,'" said Jane Good, a new grad from California who took a job as an RN on the unit she had been on all through school, "so I was glad that I had to demonstrate all my skills to my preceptor. When I 'graduated' from orientation, I got almost as much satisfaction as when I graduated from nursing school. I really know I am an equal, if inexperienced, part of the RN workforce here."

As important as how much and what kind of orientation you will have is the quality of your preceptor. It's perfectly reasonable to ask the nurse recruiter plenty of questions about how preceptors are chosen and trained. It's also relevant to ask if your preceptor has a reduced case load in the early stages of working with you, because, if not, you may have only a theoretical preceptor! Even a good intentioned and well-trained preceptor can't help double-check a vent setting if she is so overwhelmed with her patient load she barely has time to breathe herself.

In addition, you will want to know if you will be with the same preceptor for your entire orientation or if you will have a number of different preceptors. Having a few different preceptors not only makes scheduling easier but can also increase your knowledge as you get to see different ways things can be done, as well as how each nurse organizes his or her day. However, be wary of hospitals that offer only a "preceptor du jour" approach; that's when whichever nurse draws the "short straw" (or its non-metaphorical equivalent) gets to be your preceptor that shift.

How Not to Take the Nursing Shortage Personally

In this nursing shortage–stricken age, hospitals often try to deal with the decreased number of available nurses by mandating overtime, using more unlicensed assistive personnel (UAP), increasing the number of patients each nurse must take care of, and requiring nurses to float to unfamiliar units. We have seen this compared, in nursing career journals and nursing listservs and such, to "rearranging the deck chairs on the Titanic."

This is not an accurate metaphor. Studies have consistently shown that nurses leave nursing when they are forced to work mandatory overtimes, float to where they are not trained, and take care of a "nigh unto ridiculous" number of patients. So expecting these same measures to somehow relieve the nursing shortage is not like rearranging deck chairs on the Titanic, it's more like expecting the iceberg that caused the damage to the ship to magically turn into a Coast Guard cutter and ferry all the passengers to safety! It's more than futile, it's actually the anti-solution.

As a nurse—and therefore a highly sought after professional—asking about these type of issues in your initial investigation of a workplace sends a clear signal that you're interested in working in a facility committed to providing appropriate working conditions for RNs.

Use of Unlicensed Assistive Personnel

Every nurse who has been in the profession for more than a few years has an unlicensed assistive personnel horror story. These stories involve UAPs making all kinds of mistakes, from discounting a low blood sugar because the patient "seemed to be sleeping fine," to missing signs of skin breakdown, to various mishaps with feeding tubes.

It might be great to get a gig at a facility that employs an all-RN (or all-licensed) care staff, although, frankly, this also means that unless you can justify a visit from environmental services, you are almost always on your own for such fun activities as dealing with body fluids, making beds, etc. Health care economic realities being what they are, however, this situation is very rare.

Therefore, chances are you will be working with UAPs, which is not a disaster because well-trained and experienced UAPs can certainly be a valuable asset to the health-care team. The trick, then, is to get a job in a facility that makes appropriate use of UAPs. Of course, then the next challenge becomes defining what is "appropriate use" and getting accurate information from the facility about how its use compares with this definition.

The first thing you might want to do is take a gander at the American Nurses' Association statement on use of UAPs (available on their Website at nursingworld.org). The ANA statement contains some general guidelines about what types of activities may appropriately be delegated to UAPs, and also mentions some tasks that should never be delegated to UAPs, specifically anything requiring sterile technique or an invasive line. With these guidelines in mind, plan to pose some queries about the facility's use of UAPs in your initial interview. Possible ways to phrase these questions can be found in Questions to Ask About a Facility's Use of UAPs. Don't feel shy about asking! As Craig Pointer, a Pennsylvania med/surg nurse told us, "You can't go wrong bugging the nurse recruiter to provide accurate, specific information about what the people you will be supervising will be allowed to do. At worst it's your license on the line, and at the very least it will greatly affect how comfortable you feel on a day-to-day basis at work."

Questions to Ask About a Facility's Use of UAPs

What type of UAPs does this facility employ?
How are the UAPs involved in patient care (i.e., what specific tasks are they asked to complete)?
What qualifications are required for UAPs and training are they given?
How long has the average UAP been working in this facility?
How are UAPs distinguished from RNs on the unit (i.e., different color scrubs, clear designation on their ID)?

Pulling and Floating

Floating (also known as pulling, although the latter implies a slightly less voluntary nature) is not new. For example, labor and delivery nurses have been pulled to work in the new baby nursery for ages. What is relatively new is floating without cross training.

When you ask about floating practices in your interview, ask not only about the facility's policy but also about how floaters are trained and chosen (often lack of seniority is what sends you floating) and what kind of supervision and guidance is provided for you when you leave your home unit. If you are going to be floating in your orientation, ask if you get to take a preceptor along or if one will be provided at your target unit.

Mandatory Overtime

We were a little surprised (and a little scared) to read that nearly half of the nurses who responded to a 2001 ANA staffing survey, reported mandatory overtime being used to cover staffing shortages (ANA Staffing Survey, 2001). So obviously, ask if the facility requires mandatory overtime, how much notice is given if you have to work overtime, and how often (on average) this happens. It's also helpful to ask about how much voluntary overtime the average nurse at the facility works. If you are the only one on the unit not routinely working doubles so the hospital doesn't have to pay for agency nurses, that "voluntary" overtime is going to feel compulsory in no time at all.

Nurse-to-Patient Ratios

One effort being undertaken to decrease the use of the iceberg "solutions" to the Titanic problem of the nursing shortage, is mandating nurse-to-patient ratios. Most nurses we talked with thought that enacting this kind of legislation would be a positive step. However, many were skeptical about the will of hospital administrators to comply; one nurse even said, "All the mandated staffing guidelines have an 'except for public health emergencies' kind of clause. If they passed mandating staffing ratios in my state, the next day the administrators of the hospital where I work would be on the state capital steps, lobbying to have every day declared a 'public health emergency.' "

The pressure is on to pass such legislation, and a few states (led by California) have passed laws mandating either a specific ratio or that hospitals simply maintain a "safe" ratio. Of course, if acuity considerations are not written into the law and there is not some real threat of negative consequences (i.e., large fines or legal action), these laws are largely symbolic.

Hopefully, the nurse recruiter will bring up the nurse-patient ratio in your initial interview, but make sure to also ask about acuity levels and what non-RN staff would be assisting you in caring for your patients. Never, ever, ever, ever (did we mention never) be swayed or "guilted" into thinking that a desire for a reasonable nurse-patient ratio is at all related to laziness on your part. You've probably already heard about the University of Pennsylvania School of Nursing study (Aiken, 2002) that found that the odds of patient mortality in the hospital setting increased by 7% for every additional patient that a nurse is asked to care for. This is not about self-actualization, appropriate nurse-patient ratios are on the bottom of Maslow's Hierarchy of Needs, right smack dab in the middle of "safety."

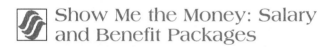

Show Me the Money: Salary and Benefit Packages

Conventional job-search wisdom maintains that it is unseemly or unprofessional for job seekers to discuss salary and benefits during the initial interview. This strikes us as an antiquated and inefficient formality. As the potential employee, unless you are living at home with mom and dad paying all the bills, you know there is a certain amount of money you have to make. The potential employer also knows there is a specific dollar amount they can afford to pay. If those amounts aren't in the same ballpark, the nurse is going to have to look elsewhere. So while it may considered "unprofessional" to mention salary in your initial interview, you increase the efficiency of the process by doing research beforehand about salary ranges in your geographical and specialty area. Talking with RN friends who have recently been scouting for jobs is a good place to start, and you can also get information about salary ranges from employment Websites (like salary.com, salaryexpert.com or payscale.com) or the U.S. Department of Labor Statistics. Of course, if you are relocating, you'll need to take into account cost of living differences when figuring out how much you need to make. The larger Web employment portals (e.g., Monster.com) offer tools for making these calculations.

When the time comes for you to ask about what kind of cold, hard, cash is available (usually in a follow-up interview, or any time after you are actually offered the job), you'll also want to ask questions about health, retirement, and education benefits. What you need or want most in a benefit package is a highly individual choice. And as you probably know from other jobs you've had, a truly exceptional benefits package can offset a low hourly wage, while a benefit package that doesn't meet your needs can be a deal breaker, no matter what kind of wads of cash the facility is offering.

Speaking of wads of cash (clever transition, ay?) let's chat a bit about sign-on bonuses. We're all adults here, we know that the bigger the sign-on bonus, the more desperate the facility is for nurses. This doesn't mean necessarily that it's a horrible place to work, only that they have, um, have a really hard time getting people to work there.

Of course, if you're a new grad and you've been eating Oodles of Noodles three times a day and buying your shoes from thrift stores for as long as you can remember, you're going to be tempted by the offer of cold, hard cash. Even those who have been working in the field awhile may be captivated by the idea of a sign-on bonus, as virtually any normal human being might. But, as Alice Grillo, a 27-year veteran of nursing told us, "Nothing comes without a price."

So if you decide to take the sign-on bonus and pay the price, it's important to know what you are committing yourself to. Inquire carefully about the terms of agreement and read the small print. What term of service are you required to complete in order to get the bonus? What happens if you are unable to complete your service or you become temporarily disabled? If you leave the job, do you have to pay the entire bonus back? Remember, in all but a very few cases, a sign-on bonus is taxable income, so your actual take-home money will be only two-thirds of the bonus amount. If you are eligible for a sign-on bonus at a place you really want to work, let us be the first to say "hooray" and invite ourselves over to your house for a lobster dinner. As Bruce Jones, a 12-year veteran nurse who now works in a pain clinic in Atlanta, Georgia, told us, "A sign-on bonus is great, as long as it's at a place a nurse is wanting to work anyway. That's what makes it a bonus, the fact that you want to work there and the extra money is the bonus." Thanks, Bruce, we couldn't have said it better ourselves.

Another factor to consider when contemplating and comparing compensation packages (how's that for alliteration!) is your eligibility for programs that assist with repayment of school loans. Some facilities offer help with loan payments in lieu of a sign-on bonus, others actually recruit students with promises of substantial payments on school loans. In addition, ask if the institution where you are applying for a job has been designated a critical shortage facility (all U.S. hospitals are now considered critical shortage facilities). If it is, the U.S. Department of Health and Human Services is now offering a program called the Nursing Education Loan Repayment Program (NELRP) just for you! If you work 2 years (at least 32 hours a week) at a participating facility, the NELRP will pay for 60% of your total loan balance, and if you work for another year, the NELRP will pay another 25% of the original loan balance. Yipee! Although not every loan is eligible for this repayment program (check out the NELRP Website at bhpr.hrsa.gov//nursing/loan-repay.htm for more details), this is a unique opportunity in that any nurse working in a critical shortage facility can apply; many hospital-based loan repayment programs are reserved for new grads.

 ## Making a Choice

Alrighty then; you had multiple interviews at Hospital A, seen the unit, met the nurse manager, investigated the facility through all human (googling them on the Web, reading their annual report) and some superhuman (calling your aunt's cousin's best friend Charlie, who once worked there) efforts. What now? Well, of course, you start all over again, completing the process with Hospitals B, C, D, and maybe even E, F, and G so you can compare and contrast their respective offers. What, you say, you've been doing that all along? Excellent. So now you're ready for the easy part of choosing which job to take.

Perhaps this is not the easy part as in "not stressful" but rather "very stressful and yet exciting." All the same, having multiple job offers to pick from is, as they say, a good thing. It may be that after your multiple tours and interviews, your choice is an obvious one. If not, you can use our handy dandy Worksheet for Comparing Job Offers to help you look at the all the various positive and negative factors for up to three jobs/facilities at once.

If you find that your decision is close, feel free to approach the recruiters at both locations to see if they have any flexibility that allows them to sweeten the deal, for example, by offering a better schedule (maybe every third weekend instead of every other), or even something small like a 1-month parking voucher.

Finally, once you've made your decision, don't forget to let the runner-up (or runners-up) know you won't be taking their job but thank you very much. And then go celebrate! You have a new job as a nurse!

 ## References

Aiken, L. H. (2002). Hospital nurse staffing and patient mortality, nurse burnout, and job dissatisfaction. *Journal of the American Medical Association,* October 23/30.

American Nurses Association. (2001). Analysis of American nurses staffing survey. Washington, DC: American Nurses' Association.

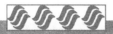

Worksheet for Comparing Job Offers

FACTOR	CONSIDERATIONS	HOW IMPORTANT IS THIS TO ME?	FACILITY NO.1	FACILITY NO. 2	FACILITY NO. 3
Institutional variation compatible with your preference?	Nonprofit vs profit? Teaching? Level one trauma center? Agency versus single facility?				
Initial orientation and preceptorship	How long is the orientation process? How are preceptors chosen and trained?				
Facility's commitment to appropriate RN working conditions	Use of UAPs? Floating? Mandatory overtime? Nurse/patient ratios?				
Salary	Is there a weekend or shift differential offered? How are raises and cost of living increases awarded?				
Sign-on bonus	How long are employees required to stay with facility after receiving the bonus? Are there any other terms or conditions?				

(continued)

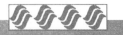

FACTOR	CONSIDERATIONS	HOW IMPORTANT IS THIS TO ME?	FACILITY NO.1	FACILITY NO. 2	FACILITY NO. 3
Educational benefits	Is continuing education provided? Tuition reimbursement? How much tuition reimbursement and over what period of time?				
Health-care benefits	Is there a waiting period before eligibility? Do employees have to pay in? How much? Are spouses, children and/or domestic partners eligible? Are dental and vision coverage also available? How comprehensive is the prescription plan?				
Sick/vacation time	How much time is provided? When does it begin to accrue? Do employees have to use time before a certain date or lose it? What are the provisions made for short-term disability?				
Specialty area	Compatible with desired specialty area?				

(continued)

FACTOR	CONSIDERATIONS	HOW IMPORTANT IS THIS TO ME?	FACILITY NO.1	FACILITY NO. 2	FACILITY NO. 3
Geographical location	Geographical location compatible with desired location?				
Commute	How long a commute? What are the commute conditions like? Is free or reduced-cost parking available? Is the facility also accessible by public transportation?				
General (subjective) feel of unit	Do staff seem relatively happy, calm, displaying effective individual coping skills? What is the state of management/RN relations?				
Schedule	Compatible with other responsibilities? Desired shift available? If desired shift is not available, how soon might you be able to change? How are weekends and holidays scheduled? Is there any flexibility in scheduling?				

(continued)

Worksheet for Comparing Job Offers (continued)

FACTOR	CONSIDERATIONS	HOW IMPORTANT IS THIS TO ME?	FACILITY NO.1	FACILITY NO. 2	FACILITY NO. 3
Retirement	What type of plans are offered? How much saving will the facility match? Is there a minimum or maximum employee contribution?				
Management/ Leadership	Does this facility help train staff nurses for management? What kinds of opportunities for advancement are available? Is the leadership style of your prospective nurse manager compatible with your personality?				

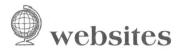 websites

About My Job
www.aboutmyjob.com
An interesting site that includes a searchable collection of job stories that details how people feel about their career and specific job choices. Fascinating and somewhat reassuring reading when you are making hard choices yourself.

All Nurses
www.allnurses.com
In lesser hands, the motto "it's how nurses surf the Web" might sound grandiose, but in this case, it's completely true. If you want real answers from real nurses to real questions you have about picking a place to work, hit this site early and often. Includes innumerable and well-organized threaded discussion boards. Recent topics included everything from are dialysis nurses paid less, to getting one's first ICU job, to what shoes to wear on a 12-hour shift. Includes posts from nurses in the United States, Canada, and a number of other countries. Also don't miss the humor section, especially the ER Math Quiz.

Center for Nursing Advocacy
www.nursingadvocacy.org
If you're interested in seeking employment at a magnet hospital, read the Center for Nursing Advocacy's section on this topic. While you're there, you can peruse the latest statistics about the nursing shortage, and read about recent issues in the media's presentation of nursing.

The Nurse Friendly
www.nursefriendly.com
This site can link the reader to anywhere on the Web it seems. Created by nurses, it contains 150,000 links in 4500 directory pages and is not restricted to solely nursing links. When looking for something particular you are able to search alphabetically, or you can browse to your heart's content and you will probably find just about anything. If you can't find the job-search information you're looking for at smaller, more specific sites, this site might come in handy.

The Nurse Village
www.nursevillage.com
If it takes a village to raise a child, it must take at least that to grow a nurse. Perhaps in that spirit, The Nurse Village offers tons of resources that can help the new grad make a decision about who should be their next employer. There is quite a bit of relocation information, including extensive articles on all aspects of major cities that are common draws for new nursing grads. Plus, you can get breaking clinical news, and send a nursing-based ecard!

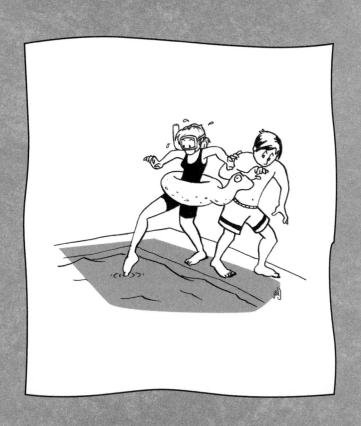

Your First Month: Dive Right In, The Water's Fine

A Nurse Speaks

My first week was very exciting and filled with much/many experiences. Unfortunately, the weeks and months following my preceptorship were very difficult. In nursing you can sink or swim; I chose to swim. I took many continuing education courses on my own to help my transition. It helps a lot to be self-motivated, that's the key to swimming.

Celeste Carangi, forensic nurse investigator

 ## Your First Day

G entleness is the key to getting through the first-day jitters. First, be gentle with yourself. Yes you, of course, need to provide safe care, but don't feel like you have to be supernurse at this moment. There will be time enough for that.

You will feel the weight of your coworkers' and manager's scrutiny upon you, but if you've gotten this far, you must be doing something right! One nurse we talked with suggested this as a first day coping strategy: "smile at people, be friendly, move quickly, and listen more than you talk." Your coworkers will probably be looking for the same thing you are looking for in a coworker—ability to "play well with others," willingness to work hard, general good-naturedness, and competency. Smiling, being friendly, and moving quickly can do an excellent job of conveying these attributes. And if you listen more than you talk, you'll learn, so that you'll be more and more competent each day!

It's important to reserve a measure of gentleness for your coworkers and the situation as a whole. Anyone can have a bad day, and the new coworker who bites your head off during report your first day might be taking care of a dying parent, dealing with an abusive spouse, etc. Of course, this kind of difficulty doesn't excuse poor behavior but sometimes the perspective alone is enough to make you want to give the person another chance. First impressions don't have to be lasting impressions if you don't hold on to them.

Also in the spirit of gentleness (and that's the last time we use that word in this chapter, promise) right after the shift (yup, stop at the dollar store on your way home) buy a notebook and write "things I do right" on the cover. Use it to record every compliment you hear about your care or attitude. Write short accounts of personal victories (the first successful IV stick on an intravenous drug user, for example) and paste in any positive notes from coworkers, patients, families, etc. It may sound juvenile, but when you have a bad day it will do your nurse-heart good to review the positive feedback you've received and milestones you've reached.

 ## Time Management

An entire book could be written about time management—okay about a bazillion books have been written about time management—but by this time in your life you've probably learned a thing or two about how to get things done in the number of minutes you are given each day. Time management in nursing—particularly in shift-based nursing—is a slightly different animal. One of the biggest differences is that you are limited in how much you can plan ahead. Part of the reason you as a nurse are present in the situation, is to deal with things that aren't planned, i.e., emergencies. So one of the biggest time-management factors, then, in shift-based nursing is completing routine tasks and responsibilities in such a way that the occasional (or frequent) unexpected event doesn't overwhelm you. In the emergency department where there are a lot of, well, emergencies, this is especially important, and so when Staci first started in the ED she developed a daily checklist she uses to organize each shift. You can find Staci's worksheet (which you can then modify as needed for your workplace) in the following box.

Many nurses cited "time management" as one of the skills they were least able to develop during nursing school. This makes sense, since

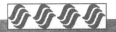

An 8-Hour Shift Organizational Checklist

This q15minute (or so) guide is geared to an emergency department setting but could be tailored to your specialty of choice or used to spark the perfect checklist of your own design:

First envision an 8-hour work shift (for the purposes of this example we are using 7 a.m. to 3 p.m.) and remember the word multitask.

0650: Arrive to work, check your hair, put the lunch you carefully prepared in the fridge. Get your diet cola or cup of coffee. Check status of unit. Quiet? Already hopping? A big mess because night shift had a crazy night?

0700: clock in (sign in)

0700–0715: Get report. Check your section of the name board. Prioritize, that is what tasks you will you be doing first. Is there an EKG needed, does someone need their blood sugar checked, are there IV antibiotic piggybacks that will soon be done and will need to be switched/come down, etc. You can write yourself a quick note next to the patient's name (on the name board) to remind yourself while you're getting report.

If you have patients, introduce yourself. While doing so, check IV fluid level statuses—you can quickly shut off almost empty piggybacks and IV bags that you will soon get back to. Eyeball your monitors: heart rhythms, b/ps, pulse ox. Eyeball your bedside supplies—suction canisters O$_2$ cannula, suction catheters, gloves in your preferred size. Can you do a quick service to show you are thinking about your patient's comfort? Say, "Are you chilly, can I get you a blanket? Would you like some water/ice chips? Do these things quick; say you'll be back soon.

0715–0730: If IV fluids need to be dealt with do that, otherwise check your code carts and fridge thermometer and test charge your defibrillators and document immediately in the appropriate book. You will quickly forget to do these things and there will be a big gaping hole where your name should be when the next nurse comes to document his/her checks. You may also need to count narcotics with another nurse at this time. Straighten up if necessary, you will feel more organized and an area looks more professional, which will make patients and their families feel more secure. Dirty linen, trash everywhere, etc., makes any unit look chaotic. Check and restock your IV supply basket or area so you're not frantically searching for stuff when you're cannulating a patient. Replace missing bedside supplies you noted earlier.

0730–0745: Do the EKGs. Document your first note per patient for the day This will usually include finding your charts, which may miraculously be in the chart rack—or more commonly you may need to wrestle them from the residents, etc. This is a quick note; the vital signs you eyeballed (go back to the monitors if necessary), patient's orientation, and if you did something—the EKG for example. You can now first check the antibiotic or other IV med orders on the ER order sheet and do those tasks. Sign off your orders immediately.

(continued)

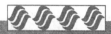
0745–0800: Fetch more coffee, place on counter, when cold—drink anyway. Check the patient's status with the ER attending; do you have any questions about the orders, who does the attending think will be getting discharged? Is the attending waiting for labs? Who will be admitted? If you can get this info, find out the admitting diagnoses, the admitting doctor, and the type of bed (telemetry, MICU, floor, etc.). You may need to get this information from the admitting team. Have they been called and are they aware of the patient's existence? How far along in the admitting process are they (are there orders written, etc.)? As soon as you have gleaned this information make sure the patient is called into registration so the nursing office/bed manager is actively looking for a bed for your patient. Remember, one of your main ER goals is to expedite the patient's speedy departure from the ER. They'll love you for it, you'll have a more effective nurse/patient ratio and you will have room for more patients. If you are lucky enough to have an ER secretary, field the calls and lab work, etc., check to them.

0800–0845: When admitting patients check if there are admitting orders and see if there is anything that needs to be done before you'll be able to send the patients to their room. Ask the admitting team if anything is urgent. Will you need to go upstairs with anyone on a monitor, if so, make a mental note. Document if you do anything. If you have a room number assigned, call the floor and request to give report. Document that you have called to do so or, if you're really lucky, document that you gave it and to which RN and when. Arrange escort to bring up the patient (or have the secretary do it). This will be a process repeated throughout the day.

This may be the time that you'll be wheeling stretchers to C/T, doing meds., IV replacement, and again checking on the status of your patients (pain levels, comfort, ADLs, etc.)

In an ER, throughout the day, you may also be receiving a new patient into an empty stretcher if you have one. How fast you will have to stop your other work in progress will depend on the severity of the presenting complaint. Even a patient that will have to wait should at least be acknowledged, directed into a gown, and given a sheet/blanket. Some will have to be immediately connected to the monitors, O_2, etc. Your triage nurse usually will field this but he/she may need your immediate assistance if the situation is urgent.

The triage person will also do the initial documentation of vital signs and history. If it's busy, this beginning process can be repeated multiple times and will obviously take a large amount of time. Flexibility is a must, but always temper your decision with the concept of what is the priority for a patient's safety, maintenance of medical stability, and then expedition of the admission process, in that order. A new patient may have to wait if an already present patient is in clinical trouble, or an old patient might have to wait if a new patient arrives in fulminant pulmonary edema. You will quickly realize your priorities in these cases.

(continued)

For example, a skeleton urgent new patient management scenario: cardiac or otherwise unstable patient: 1. Undress, IV line, monitor, O_2 (simultaneously you will be assessing vital signs, respiratory status, any history from the paramedics, family, pt., etc. Start thinking about the possible causes of the patient's trouble); 2. EKG; and 3. Ask the ER doc about what meds, IV fluids. Obtain them and administer and document as soon as you can, at patient's bedside if necessary. You may be working with the triage nurse or other nurses in an emergent situation and all of these things may happen almost simultaneously.

0845–1400: Repeat directives from 0730–0845 Mix well and don't forget to drink water. Remember, you should never wait until the end of the day to document. Document per task if possible. Document if there's a vital sign/mental status/pain level/disposition/, etc., change. You won't be able to remember times or some specifics if you let too many hours go between notes. It will also be an added stressor over your head that you won't need.

Keep the patients and their families informed. This can be a quick, "We got a room for you, it's No. 236" or, "The orthopedic doctor is in OR but will be down as soon as he can be," or, "I didn't forget that you're hungry, I ordered you lunch," etc. Patients more than anything want to know what is going on and that you know they still exist. They need to know that you have them on your mind. You know you do, but as you trot by, their anxiety level is rising and they will take it out on you because there is no one else to take it out on. You will have a calmer day overall if you manage these kinds of simple interactions.

If you have down time, can't move patients upstairs because you're waiting for XYZ, etc., and everyone is stable and as comfortable as possible:

- Eat something (preferably not a candy bar)
- Check your nurse compatriots. Is anyone drowning and in need of assistance?

1400: Start thinking about the shift ending. Do final notes (an emergent patient may need one almost at the change of shift). Since you have been documenting all day these should be vital signs and a quick final eval, not a six paragraph dissertation. Think back to your 0700 activities. Are your IV fluids that are hanging OK? Can you do any last minute tasks to make the patient comfortable or to lessen the load on the next shift? Do you need to restock anything? If you're very busy, start thinking priority again and make a mental note about what will be the things you must pass on to the next shift as the most urgent to do. If at all possible, make another attempt to give report on your admitted patients, as you know them best, even if they will not be able to go up until next shift. You may have time for a bathroom break now—or not.

And finally, remember, that before you even realize it, this and other unit and facility processes are going to become like breathing to you. You will be assessing people in the neighborhood diner and you'll be remembering six patients' full vital signs in your head perfectly before you even know it. You are going to feel competent and like a true advocate for your patients and it's going to feel good. Nursing gets into your pores because of the very nature of the importance of it. Don't worry, you'll see.

nursing school clinicals are seldom 8 hours long, let alone 12, and nursing students even in their last year seldom carry a full patient load. Thus, even if you had a lot of varied experiences, opportunities to try procedures, etc., during your clinical experiences, you can't expect that school prepared you for the real world of floor nursing. Hopefully, your nurse manager, and coworkers will realize this and not expect superhuman results (even though you are probably exerting superhuman effort). In the meantime, heed the words of Jill Hall, a California RN, "If you find you're getting behind ask for help sooner rather than later. Prioritize constantly. There are days when you will have to let the less important items go undone. It's really difficult to transition from the perfect standards taught in nursing school to real world situations. Remember that in school each procedure involved all the time in the world, all the equipment and help you needed plus a cooperative patient. It rarely happens that way. In reality you do the best job you can with what you've got, aiming for the highest possible standards."

 ## Surviving Shift Work

If you've ever been around anyone who is chronically fatigued, you know it can be a trying experience for you because it is such a very trying experience for them. Kelli took a number of her RN-BSN classes with nurses who worked the night shift, and at least one admitted, "I've been tired for the last 20 years. I don't know what it's like to not be tired." These were (usually) women with child-related responsibilities during the day, or dads who worked a second job. The fact that they managed to study, let alone be safe when driving or working could only be attributed to a series of small miracles, perhaps arranged by the patron saint of night-shift workers, whoever that is. Regardless of their success, being habitually tired is not just a discomfort issue. We're nurses, we know that chronic fatigue leads to illness, decreased resistance to stress, decreased immune function, and also impaired cognitive abilities. And doesn't this sound like something a nurse might want to avoid?

"Unless you are one of the few naturally nocturnal of our species, when you work night shift you are basically going against your total biology," pointed out Haley Brown, an Iowa RN, "so be prepared to work for your sleep." How do you do this? The most important action to take is make sleep a priority, and then, perhaps even more importantly, communicate this. "Your family and friends can't assume that you can 'sleep anytime,' but they will if you have that kind of attitude," said Margaret Oslo, a Philadelphia ED nurse. "You need to have set, predetermined sleeping times. And one day if you find you can't sleep during those times, hide out! Never talk to anyone or let any of your friends/

family see you when you're supposed to be sleeping because then they will come to think of it as optional and always feel like they can interrupt you if they deem it important. This is especially true of kids."

Besides having a set schedule (which may be nigh unto impossible due to rotating shifts), other nurses have found that adaptation to the night shift can be facilitated by the use of earplugs during the day, an established going-to-sleep ritual, use of aromatherapy (a few drops of lavender essential oil on the pillow, for example), and avoidance (gulp!) of caffeine (certainly much easier said than done).

Despite the difficulties in adjusting to a nocturnal lifestyle, many nurses enjoy some of the unique benefits and challenges that come with working nights. Celeste Carangi, a forensic nurse investigator with years of ED experience, said, "I enjoy night shift. That's the most satisfying shift for me. It can be difficult because you have less support in house at night, but you need to be more autonomous and creative. In the long run it helps you to be more assertive and a more independent person." See Jen Borek's A New Grad Speaks for her introduction to shift work.

Night shift is not the only shift work–related challenge nurses face. A 3-to-11 shift can be difficult, but usually for a different reason— decreased social interaction. "I started out second shift when I was out of school and I liked it because I could still go out late with my friends and then sleep in," said a Brooklyn-based ICU nurse, "but when I got married and had kids I didn't like that schedule anymore. My husband was supportive, but I still felt like I was missing the best hours with my children. Of course, when they were school-age they liked that I was available to go to their homerooms or see their school plays during the day. I felt like it was even more urgent to be around as they got older. One day I read an article about teen pregnancy and it said that most teen pregnancies are conceived between 3 p.m. and 5 p.m., in other words, in between the time kids get home from school and parents come home from work. Within an hour I applied to change to 7 a.m. to 3 p.m." One way of mitigating the effect second shift can have on family and social life is to have pre-set lunch arrangements with family and friends, for example, every Thursday you meet your best friend for lunch, and you schedule family lunches together whenever the kids are out of school (including on weekends).

Another difficult aspect of shift work is working holidays and weekends when others are off. Although most nurses eventually adapt to this part of the nurse lifestyle, it can be hard, especially at first. Many nurses said their families grew to understand that they would be working holidays and would try hard to create rituals that could fit into their working schedule. For example, one nurse who works nights said her family now does a big (and early) Christmas eve dinner and then they open presents when she returns home at 7 a.m. on Christmas day.

Monday, June 30, 2003

Tonight was my first night on 11 to 7. I tried to nap before I went in but I couldn't sleep. I am due in at 10:45 p.m. for report. I went to Wawa for coffee and packed a lunch. I got there a little early, and met the other nurses. I am now paired with Kathie, a terrific nurse who has been there for a few years. The floor where I am assigned is two north. 2N is a 15 bed floor of private rooms. This is where the patients with TB, MRSA, or any other special precautions go. It is also the floor with the suctioning and the vents. For this part of my orientation, I am going to be trained on primary care. Kathie and I have half of the patients on the floor. She and I take report and make rounds. We provide all of the patient care but not meds, there is a charge/meds nurse. One of our patients required a lot of care and a lot of suctioning. He had a nasal trumpet. I had never seen one before, let alone suctioned from one. All I could do was watch. It was the sound more than the sight. When Kathie was suctioning out the patients mouth, she pulled out what looked like a liver. That was it, I had seen enough. I threw out my dinner. As the night went on, I was surprised that I was not really tired. It was a strange feeling driving home at that time of day. I went right to bed and slept until 2 p.m.

Tuesday, July 1, 2003

Tonight I am back on 2N. I had a patient on a ventilator. The vent was supplementing the patient's own breaths and keeping her at a set rate per minute. I learned the settings and how to record the information on the vent sheet. Often times an alarm would sound for one reason or another. Each time I would go to the room and check. Usually before I got to the door it would stop. One time it didn't. As I got to the room the machine read APNEA, I thought, oh my God, she's coding. I looked at her and she was taking some breaths, what was wrong? The other nurse calmly came in and reconnected the vent to her trach. I felt like an idiot, how could I have missed something so obvious. The patient was fine and we had a good laugh at my panic.

Wednesday, July 2, 2003

Tonight was my first night suctioning. I had a patient on a vent with inline suctioning. It was not too bad. I still am not able to eat while I'm at work though. This could [be] one diet I really stick to.

Thursday, July 3, 2003

I am getting into a routine with my assessments, flow sheets, treatments, I&Os etc. I really like nights. I am not tired until I leave, and I am able to fall asleep right when I get home. The kids are really behaving. I have been getting up a little earlier so we can go to the pool. I try to lie down around 7:30 for a nap before I go in. It's working so far.

(continued)

Friday, July 4, 2003

The hospital was short for 3 to 11 shift so I offered to come in. I worked on 2N again. I feel really comfortable on that floor. I am even able to suction without a problem. Changing the canister still grosses me out though! It was a quiet night and I am looking forward to the weekend.

Monday, July 7, 2003

I had a nice weekend catching up on some things around the house. I was assigned primary care on 2N. Nothing too eventful. I am looking forward to training for charge nurse later this week.

Tuesday July 8, 2003

Tonight I am on 4S, the med-surg orthopedic floor with Kathie training to be charge nurse. We are responsible for all of the meds and the chart checks. We make sure the IV fluids are correct and infusing. We prepare any patients for surgeries before 9 a.m.. In addition we admit any patients to the unit. Tonight there were three admissions. The ER was busy and the hospital was flooded with admissions. Just as I would finish the assessment for one patient, the ER would call with report on the next. We were so busy. The night flew by.

Wednesday, July 9, 2003

Tonight we are back on 4S in charge. It was a much quieter night and we spent a lot of time going over all of the things that the charge nurse is responsible for. I am really learning so much. I don't know how I'll ever keep it straight. Luckily, I am paired with a wonderful preceptor who is really teaching me so much.

Thursday, July 10, 2003

Before I went to nursing school, I took a phlebotomy course. The main part of my last job was drawing blood. This made me interested in starting IVs. We had a one day course in nursing school. I always watch the IV team put in IVs. I know it's silly, but I think I would be good at it. Tonight, one of the patients needed a restart. They called the IV nurse to start a new line. When I asked to watch he said, why don't you do it? So I did. He walked me through it and I got it. I was so excited.

Friday, July 11, 2003

Tonight I was back on 2N doing primary care. It was a pretty uneventful night until my morning I&O rounds. My patient had only put out 5cc from his Foley. I checked him and the Foley was in, but leaking. I checked the size, it was 14fr. I went and got another kit, a 16fr this time. It was just like in school. I put in the Foley and when I saw urine in the tube I advanced it, inflated the balloon, and as I was pulling back urine started spraying all over the place from around the tubing. I was so shocked and yet I never broke sterile technique or let go of his penis. The other nurse was hysterical laughing and said "Jen, you can let go, you can let go." We both were hysterical after that. I then inserted an 18 fr which was a better fit. Thankfully, the patient slept through the whole thing.

As for how you feel about working holidays and weekends, try to reframe the situation if you can. Shift work means that sometimes you are working when others are playing, but this also means sometimes you are off when others are working. Because of this, you can take your kids to the amusement park on weekdays during the summer when it's cheaper and less crowded and you can run your errands on a weekday morning before bank and grocery store are mobbed.

 ## Uniforms and Equipment

"I didn't buy anything new when I set foot in my first hospital job," said Brian French, a Louisiana new grad, "I found that they required us to buy so much stuff in nursing school—most of which I never used—that I was more than adequately equipped for the first 2 years." Many of the nurses we talked with echoed this sentiment, with one very notable exception, shoes.

In nursing school, even if you had clinical as often as three times a week, you simply were not spending as much time on your feet as you will be at your first nursing job. Adequate footwear—in fact, the very best that you can afford—will save not only your feet, but also your hips, knees, and back. Shoes made for nurses are always good (did you know the first woman to run the Boston Marathon did so in nurses' shoes because no women's running shoes were available at the time), but you can also go to your friendly neighborhood footwear retailer and talk to the staff there. Although it will definitely be more expensive if you go to a place with trained staff who can look at your stride and evaluate what kind of shoe is best for you, it will definitely be worth it. Beware, though, of the super-lightweight running shoes that have uppers made almost entirely of canvas mesh. Although they will feel very light, they won't adequately protect your feet. Of course, short of wearing combat boots encased in concrete (which would, of course, cause another set of problems) nothing can totally protect your tootsies. However, it doesn't feel nearly as bad when a dislodged supply cart rolls over your foot when you're wearing a sturdy leather shoe rather than a dainty little high-tech canvas mesh number. If you can afford to buy a few pairs of shoes, so much the better. It will give your shoes a chance to really air out between wearings, which drastically increases the life of the shoes and also makes them a lot more pleasant, olfactorily speaking.

You might also want to invest in a few more pair of work-only socks. You may have noticed other folks' body fluids have a mysterious way of seeking socks, so white is best, so you can bleach them. An extra stethoscope can also come in handy, as well as your own BP cuff. Frankly, now that people know you're a nurse, you're probably going to get a lot of "can you check Aunt Millie's pressure? She has a terrible headache" type requests.

Finally, buy pens in bulk. You're going to lose them, give them away, abandon them secondary to body fluid contamination, have them stolen by residents, etc.

As for uniforms, if your employer supplies your "Lollydwaggle University Hospital" scrubs, there's not a whole lot to say here. If not, mail order and/or online scrubs can be a good deal and make it easier to find the desired size and color (once you've ordered once and know what size you need), but beware of the cheapest of cheap scrubs. Kelli ordered some of the "super special bargain" scrubs from a certain well-known nursing mail order company and found they were so thin she was embarrassed to wear them anywhere but bed.

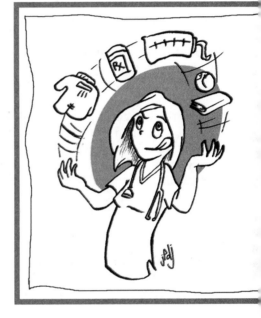

We also talked with a number of nurses who made their own scrubs. Yes, made them, meaning sewed them together from scratch out of cloth. Neither of us are so Martha Stewartesque (even postconviction) to attempt something like this, but apparently many nurses are. Actually since scrubs are relatively cheap, it's usually more expensive to make them from scratch, but as one nurse said, "I like making the scrubs to fit me just right and I also like having more material options. I also like knowing I can put a pocket where I want it, not where the scrub manufacturers think it should be."

Finally, you may want to invest some money into references for your new job, particularly if you are in a new specialty area. Many books are available in electronic format for your PDA (for example, F.A. Davis has many different titles available, including the useful for new grads *RN Notes* as well as their drug reference and *Taber's Medical Dictionary*), so be sure to check into that option if you'd like avoid lugging heavy books around. If you're unsure about the potential usefulness of any reference, check it out on amazon.com or book-sense.com (the independent bookseller's Web presence). Not only will you find user reviews, but both sites offered detailed information about books and sometimes even allow you to download (or at least peruse) a sample chapter.

Resources

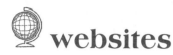 websites

Medilexicon
www.medilexicon.com
Ever stood at the nurses' station wondering what "patient is KLOKM, was able to FIKL × 2 during TYRW," means? It's a typical new-grad problem. You can use this site—which explains more than 140,000 medical abbreviations—to figure out such things. Has both a Spanish and English version. The site is free to use, and for a small fee you can download a version for your personal digital assistant.

Notes on ICU Nursing
www.icufaq.com
What an amazing resource! Written by Mark Hammerschmidt and Jayne Mulholland, two nurses with almost 40 years of ICU experience between them, this site contains a series of responses to frequently asked questions about working in the ICU. Although somewhat particular to the hospital where they work, these documents are so amazingly detailed, down-to-earth, and well written, they are potentially useful for any new grad or new transfer to the ICU. Start by reading the section called The New RN in the MICU. The documents are in MS Word form and are in the public domain so you can download and share them with your new-grad friends and coworkers.

Rich Dad, Poor Dad Online
www.richdadpoordad.com
Unfortunately, financial education has never been considered part of the three "Rs" (maybe because "financial" starts with an "f?") and so many of us could use a little help in understanding how to create a workable financial plan. This site, created by Robert T. Kiyosaki (author of *Rich Dad, Poor Dad: What the Rich Teach Their Kids About Money That the Poor and Middle Class Do Not*, and many other titles) provides a whole new way of looking at finances. The basic tenets (develop passive income and stop working for someone else) are not exactly rocket science; it's the engaging and simple way Kiyosaki presents them that has bazillions of people buying his books. While breaking completely free from the "rat race" (i.e., working for someone else) isn't really practical for everyone (what are nurses going to do, open our own hospitals? Hmmm…), the plethora of information here is still quite useful. You can download sample chapters of all Kiyosaki's books as well as try a demo of the electronic Cash Flow Game, or participate in the threaded discussion boards (requires free registration to post).

The Sleep Foundation's Shiftwork Suggestion Site

www.sleepfoundation.org/publications/shiftwork.cfm

This site contains suggestions for maintaining your health and sanity while doing shift work. Includes tips on successful sleeping, balancing life and work, staying awake during the drive home, and ways to promote alertness at work (besides a 1:12 nurse-patient ratio).

The Student Nurse Forum

http://kcsun3.tripod.com

Well, it's true that you're no longer a student, but you'll find this site useful just the same. You can review basic courses, secure continuing education credits, and learn more about time management on the floor. You can also send your fellow new grads an ecard that says congrats on their first week at work. They're free, so send one to yourself, too!

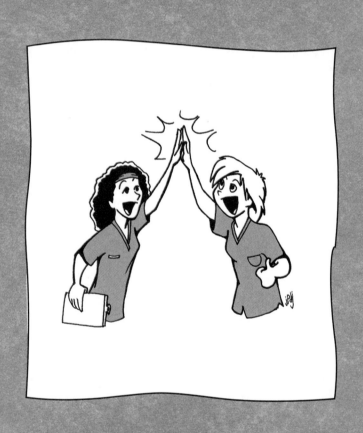

Fostering Healthy Relationships

A Nurse Speaks:

The relationships you have with your coworkers are what makes or breaks the work environment. If you feel that you can't work as a team with your peers, or that you can't ask for help without a backlash, you're going to be frustrated and miserable. This in turn can affect your behavior with patients, even though you don't want it to. On the other hand, when there is open communication, camaraderie, and a feeling of "we're in this together, I've got your back!" you feel you can surmount even the most stressful or difficult work experience. When the unit works together smoothly the patients notice. They also notice when there is sniping or negativity. This increases their anxiety and stress level and believe me, you'll be the one having to deal with it! I've been told more than once over the years by patients and families alike, that the efficient, calm, good-humored way the nurses on my unit work together puts them at ease. It makes them feel that we're professionals with a strong handle on the situation and the tools to help them through their most difficult times. So, the patients feel more relaxed and their reactions make us feel great—capable and even more invested in working together. It really does become a positive cycle!

D.R., SICU RN, New Jersey, 16-year veteran.

⚕ Family and Friends in a Time Of Transition

During the stressful time of beginning a new nursing position, it's very easy to forget about the people in the rest of your life (and yes, you will have a "rest of your life"). Even though you'll be caught up with trying to gain control of some kind of logical sleeping and eating regimen, managing your time and emotional resources, and trying to refrain from talking about difficult Foley placements or DSM IV diagnoses, your need for "your people" and their need for you will still be a constant. When asked what new and returning nurses could do to maintain good relationships with family and friends during this beginning crunch time, this is what some of the nurses we interviewed had to say:

- "...Discussing with them [family and friends] PRIOR to starting the job about how busy your really going to be. Dividing up household responsibilities, eliciting support from extended family for help. Then making time for family and understanding that it's going to be hard for them. Eventually it slows down and life returns to normal." Regina Moore, Emergency Dept., Trauma Coordinator RN, 11-year veteran, Colorado.
- "...Recognizing that the new nurse is not the only one in transition— the family and friends have new challenges too." Alice Grillo, Operating Room, Orthopedics RN, 27-year veteran, Pennsylvania.
- "Encourage open communication!" Arlena Williams, Emergency Dept. RN, 7-year veteran, Pennsylvania
- "Put aside time for the family (as in *schedule* time) until routines are set." Molly Raimondi, Emergency Dept. RN, 31-year veteran, Pennsylvania
- "A difficult question indeed. Ensure that your family understands you're under great pressure and may be tired/moody. Don't schedule overtime shifts, you need your family and relaxation time." Jill Hall, Pediatric ICU RN, 3-year veteran, New Jersey.
- "Talk about what's going on with your new job—your feelings, expectations, etc." Diane Wench, Emergency Dept. RN, 27-year veteran, Pennsylvania.

Hopefully you're picking up a theme here—open communication. Many others, especially concise nurse interviewees, replied to this question by simply saying only that, "Communicate!" (As a little side game you may want to count how many times you see this word in this book.

E-mail us with the correct number of times and we'll send you a prize or, at least a commendation for your tenacity!)

Everyone reacts to change, even positive change. As a rule, when people are informed, they are more able to mentally prepare and do not react as oppositionally when it occurs. And just as in the medical world, certain groups are more fragile or susceptible to changes in their environment. Your young children (2 to 7 year olds) will need frequent (daily at first), simple updates on what's going to change, e.g., when your time with them will be, who's going to pick them up from school or play groups, who will be reading to them at night and putting them to bed, where you are when your not with them, and assurance you can be reached if it's an emergency; why your new work is important and necessary; and most importantly, *frequent reassurance* (try five times a day and whittle it down) that you love them as much as always and you always will, even when your grumpy or tired. If you can keep your young children's daily routines as consistent as possible, their stress level will be less escalated and this will benefit you, too. On days off, try to start a special, simple, one-on-one tradition and stick with it, such as an hour of time reading and drawing together, or baking together, bike riding together, singing together, 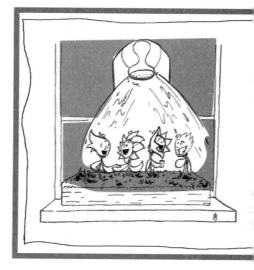 and so on (age appropriate, of course). Your children will come to look forward to this and see it as a positive consequence of your new career. This will also benefit you as a centering, stabilizing force in the (probably) hectic, anxiety-producing schedule you have adopted of late. The most important part of this is to keep these plans *simple*—don't promise the kids you'll take them to the amusement park every Tuesday or start a softball league—and then, (did I mention this?) stick to the plan. And yes, if you're not going to be there for a bedtime, definitely give a brief goodnight call from your job (you can fit in one more "I love you" then).

Your teenagers, although—or perhaps because—they are more physically self-sufficient pose other challenges. It has been statistically shown that many older kids get into most of their "trouble" during the time frame of after-school to 8 p.m. One benefit of nursing is our glorious early start time for day shift—usually 7 a.m. This can get you home in time to start your second full-time job of childrearing, etc. Of course, there will be shift rotation or possibly 12-hour shifts, etc., and, as Staci, who has two daughters ages 14 and 15, can attest, child management will always be an issue and will have to be planned for. Teenagers generally won't tell you that they want or need supervision—au contraire! They are, nevertheless, capable of showing you their resentment in myriad ways. Acting out, declining school grades, increased testing of your authority, and other pleasantries may ensue. Thanks to their increased autonomy, they will be called on to make more and more of their own decisions. This, of course, is a hallmark of adolescence, and completely necessary for development. In the absence of an acceptable level of parental involvement however, these decisions may contain an unacceptable level of error or danger. So what to do? Mandatory family times should be, well, mandatory. Again, this should be simple "just be together" time. If it comes down to a few meals together per week then make them count. Demand no TV, check school work, practice guitar together, listen to your kid's CDs with him or her, etc. In essence make your presence known. They may balk (we mean they will balk—it's their job!) but they do need and want your caring and supervision. You can also demand that some of their friend/social activity occurs under your roof when you're home, or in some area where you can eye, er...meet their friends and get a feel for what your kid's peers are into. And, your entire family should have a plan set up if there is an emergency of the peer-pressure kind. This could involve drinking and driving, and any other dangerous activity you (and hopefully your kids) want to avoid. You can and should set up and even role-play (yes, we did say role play) various scenarios beforehand. It could be one of those together-dinner's topics of conversation. Your adolescent should be able to call you, and/or other designated persons (you'll definitely need backup—remember the 12-hour shifts?) and, if necessary, sound very surly, angry, etc., about having to do it. They then can very unhappily but resolutely inform their compatriots that they have to stay where they are and not get in the drunk person's car, or finish with the pushy boy's date, etc., because, "My mom/dad, etc., is such a so and so, and I'm in big trouble, and ENTER APPROPRIATE TALL-TALES HERE" (reform/military school, etc.). When they call, maybe one specific curse word would be used—one that you normally would not EVER hear coming out of your child's mouth (at least not connected to you in any way), or some other logical "code" word could be utilized to convey the urgency of the situation. It should be made very clear, that under no circumstances should this code word or call-scenario take place as a joke (invoke the boy who cried wolf at this time). At Staci's house, one hilarious "scenario drill" ended up with a code about taking the cat to the vet.

This was ditched due to impracticality, but you get what we mean. An important aspect of this "escape plan" is that your adolescent knows he/she can call even if they have done something wrong (say, drank alcohol) and you or your designees will still get them and not immediately (no, we didn't say never) begin berating them. Of course, wrong actions still carry consequences, but the fact that your teen has trusted you and ultimately made a good decision should count for a lot. It takes a lot of bravery for a youth to say no, even with help, and this should be sincerely considered. Now, if this occurs every Saturday night, you'll have some serious counseling and game planning and, possibly grounding, to do, but at least you'll have them safe and home to do it. This code set-up has several benefits. A prepared plan circumvents panic for your teen (which always causes poor judgment calls). Your expectations are clear from the get-go, and probably most importantly, you are sending a message to these, hard to-get-through-to humans that you care, that you're there for them even if you're doing this intense job called nursing.

In connection with this, and in our modern world, a cell phone for your kids probably would be appropriate. Especially if your teens go straight to extra-curricular activities after school or if they work, and so on. May we suggest pre-paid phone cards, not programs that allow your kids to run up lovely $500 phone bills for the family plan! And speaking about activities, etc., you should know what the weekly schedule is (and your kids should know yours). You should expect check-in calls at predetermined times, and that includes where you nurse. Parents abound in nursing and we have never heard of anyone getting flack from managers about someone's child giving an "I'm OK" call to a parent at work. If you absolutely can't get to the phone when they call, call them back ASAP. And, if it's at all possible, have a conscientious neighbor check in. Maybe have your teens and their friends rotate in (small) groups to where a parent might be home after school. The idea is cultivating the "eyes in the back of your head" routine.

If this sounds like a lot more stress and planning and preparation and calling and... just think about if you have to react to a catastrophe, or if you find out about a problem a little too late. You will be much calmer and therefore more able to focus on mastering your chosen profession if you proact instead of react.

As for the adult significant others in your life, in the beginning (or maybe forever), it can be helpful to make actual, written down dates for time together. You'll be amazed at how the weeks will slide by without you and yours having any "quality time" together. Of course, this can be dates for dining and dancing, but you will also crave simple, grounding activities, such as time gardening or reading to each other, walking, attending your chosen religious ceremony together, etc. And don't forget the importance of home time. We're not talking about, "Dear, you clean the downstairs toilet and I'll clean the upstairs toilet." We mean cooking and having a meal together and playing footsie on the couch, etc. (NOT with the TV on)! Just taking the time to plan and demanding these time slots conveys that you intend to keep your loved ones a priority. It will also give you something to look forward to on the inevitable days of high stress and low emotional return.

And keep in mind our catch phrase (you know, right?) communication. Ask for help, ask for an extra boost, ask for a back rub, ask for pizza night on your 4th 12-hour shift in a row, even if it falls on your traditional "3-hour beef brisket and homemade pie" night (or maybe someone else can make the 3-hour brisket!). Maybe your best buddies can come over to your home and play Parcheesi and "kibbitz" a bit when you're exhausted from your new role instead of partying down and boogying all night like you "always" did on Saturday nights. (We have a feeling nursing school may have already knocked a little bit of this out of you already.)

It is very important to remember and frequently remind yourself that it is not weakness to ask for help, but an actual strength; a strength that will allow you to excel in your nursing as well as other areas of life. It will allow you to have the emotional and physical wherewithal to not just survive your new job and juggle your family and friends, but actually enjoy all of these things. If you don't communicate your needs, your personality will show the strain, and you and the people who love you will feel isolated and frustrated. But with an open dialogue, this time of transition can be a time of self-discovery and growth.

Patients and Their Families

We now want to address one of the most important and difficult areas of daily nursing life—the delicate subject of the care and feeding of the general public. Nurses are certainly deliverers of health care. We save lives, help to cure illness, and so on. What is as true and many times more imperative is our role of ambassador, counselor, mediator, emotional support, and patient advocate. Because of the environment we work in, this does not boil down to just being sympathetic and kind, although these qualities do play a role.

We'll discuss our interaction with patients and their families in two parts.

First, we'll discuss patients. Patients—as you are already well aware—are why we are nurses. We have signed on specifically to care for people.

We want to help them. The question will be, how to do this in their best interest. If all it took were being nice, it would be easy. The reality is that patients will want to do things that are counterproductive to recovery. This could be not using their incentive spirometer or continuing cutting behaviors, or practicing wanton polypharmacy or ripping their IVs out to go have a cigarette in the bathroom. The list of how patients can sabotage their own health is endless and ranges from pathologic to just natural human inclination. Many times it's related to lack of knowledge not purposeful obstreperousness.

You will be amazed at how often you would not be able to call yourself a patient advocate if you give a patient what he or she wanted. This can go all the way to having damaging legal or licensure ramifications in the more extreme contexts.

So what's a poor nurse to do? Well, first we have to recognize that there is a balance that must be attained. We are not a patient's buddy but we are not their mothers or drill sergeants either. We have to come around to a realization of what our role is and then, each of us must personally find a way to congenially, professionally, and consistently convey this to our clients. So what is our role? We've mentioned deliverer of health care and patient advocate to name two. In the delivery of health care (and we realize we're just skimming the surface) we are to carry out a doctor's orders with a vigilant eye on contraindications to those orders. We are to monitor, with all of our senses, mental capacity, and training, a patient's physical and mental state throughout our time of interaction, and any and all reactions, positive and negative, to abovementioned orders. We are to use nursing skills to prevent or minimize adverse effects of illness. This could be positioning and ADL care, reorientation, aspiration precautions, or providing a calm, quiet environment to name a few of a thousand.

As far as giving meds and being the watchdog for physician errors, med allergies, and calculating drug delivery rates, we think you will be able to be vocal and firm in your convictions. A wrong med or a dropping blood pressure is a concrete thing and there's no nebulousness about what course of action must be taken. It is when we talk about nursing care to minimize the effects of illness that things can get a little sketchy. The action taken to fulfill this statement will be different depending on the context. It can even be contradictory at times. What do we mean? There will be times when you will need to gauge risk/benefit ratios. Is the patient so humiliated by residual from a CVA, that forcing him to have a bed bath (albeit safer and probably more thorough and definitely faster) instead of somehow arranging assistance for him in the shower or bathroom, or even clumsily at bedside, will hinder healing rather than support it? Or conversely, when would a bed bath, even if not totally necessary, be the nurturing experience that causes a person to feel valued enough to want to go on living? These considerations will also have to be assessed with your total patient load and the acuity level du jour as well.

This part of patient relations is the more subjective part. We, as nurses, must somehow juggle patient dignity and free will with what is going to produce the most positive health outcome. By law, we are not allowed to force medical care or any physical touch or treatment upon any individual. This rule is amended at times when patients are medically determined to not be able to make sound decisions for themselves by virtue of mental illness, drug effects and/or other mind-altering circumstances. But even during an event when it is determined that physical restraints are necessary (We interrupt this sentence to just say...document.), we still must try and remember what is most important to our patients. This knowledge must be the basis from which all our decisions related to patient relations must spring. All patients want to be treated as important. All patients want to be treated as individuals. All patients want not to suffer unnecessarily. All patients want to get the optimum level of care available. If our interactions with our patients are guided by these facts, we then must figure out how to convey that we know this. Well, if we are talking to a friend or coworker we use eye contact. This should be so with patients as well. Don't walk by people without some recognition of their existence, whether in a hall or office or bed.

It's also important to become aware of differences in acceptable ways to address people in different age groups. Don't call elderly people "baby" or "sweetie" or the like. Keep in mind that we, too, will be old one day and will not want to be infantilized. It's a good rule to use Mr. or Mrs. So and So for at least most initial conversation (probably not with a 10-year-old, though).

It can be challenging, but it's helpful to remember cultural differences when interacting with patients and their families. Otherwise one can easily dismiss someone's behavior as melodrama or at the other end of the spectrum—indifference/apathy. In reality, what you may be witnessing is the cultural norm for that specific group. Different reactions to illness, death, family dynamics, etc., are encoded in our upbringings and cultural experiences. What is seen as common decency and polite interaction in, let us say, the African-American community in Philadelphia, could be considered intrusive or rude in the Korean community, and vice-versa. Our own personal reactions are guided by our cultural and ethnic backgrounds as well. Our professional reactions, though, must err on the side of conscious judgment, as snap-judgment leads to minimizing our patients worth, stereotyping, and sometimes leads to inappropriate (or at least not optimal) treatment modalities. So, allow people to give you their own story in their own way. Sometimes, you'll have to redirect them or their train of thought back toward what information you're trying to elicit, but at least let patients give some background or let them express their fear, anxiety, or concerns before that redirection.

Never speak to someone else over a patient as if he or she is not there—always include or explain to the patient what you're saying, etc. You want to convey that you consider the person an equal, someone able to understand information. This leads us to a key way we convey worth to our patients. Clear, concise patient teaching not only affects patient outcome, it makes people feel you actually care about their getting and staying better. Write down precise, simple directives (e.g., "Increase your fluid intake, noncaffeinated drinks—at least 8, 10-oz. glasses a day. You can use popsicles or soup, as well"). Write down follow-up appointment dates with office phone numbers, and any medications, their dosage schedules, and possible major side effects or contraindicated food/meds. Use large print.

Read everything you wrote out loud to the patient and watch for recognition or confusion. Use any opportunity during care to discuss the things a patient might expect, or be concerned about. As JD, a 35-year veteran told us about her experience in patient teaching, "I figure if I explain things 3 times, I've just gotten started. Repetition is key. Patient teaching is a must whether you're in a patient's home, hospital room, or obstetrics office. As a matter of fact, patient teaching is one of the tools that nurses use that make us professionals rather than skilled-based laborers.

Many institutions have preprinted instruction/discharge sheets, but we have come to find that patients can become intimidated by small print and a lot of it. They may not even attempt to read it, or not thoroughly. Of course, still give the patient the information (with the most pertinent areas circled, etc.) but add handwritten directives as mentioned. This, as well as your verbal reinforcement, will be what most patients will rely on.

Relations with a patient's family are directed by the same common-sense guidelines. Most nurses we talked with agreed that it's very important to a patient's significant others that they be allowed to be an advocate (for example, by providing background information), that they are kept as up-to-date as possible (bear in mind the patient has a right to not have information disseminated, definitely ask first), and especially, that they be allowed to be *with* the patient as much as possible.

When we're extremely busy (which, of course, we almost always are) we can sometime slip into behavior that might convey to the family the attitude that they are a hindrance to performance of care or are adversaries, or the cause of all the patient's problems. But this adds unnecessary stress to the patient's environment and to your own! You will get just the adversaries you conjured up. On the other hand, if families come at you in defensive mode, this is easily diffused or at least restructured by using the methods discussed to convey that you recognize the family's worth and importance.

Nursing school curriculum addresses relationships with patients but most nurses we talked with said they got little instruction about dealing with families. One new grad said, "I realize our concern is focused on the patient, but the more experience I get, the more I am convinced that we are treating the family too. Did nursing school cover what to do, for example, when the family is fighting around you while you're trying to check an IV? Nope, and if that kind of thing happened in clinical, it was usually the primary nurse who took care of it. I work on an oncology floor and the families are usually in shock and/or grieving and are also very involved. It's been difficult to learn the delicate balance between keeping the family involved and making sure the patient doesn't feel left out in the confusion! I also had to come to the somewhat painful realization that we aren't going to make all families happy. Someone they love is dying...why would they be? Sometimes we bear the brunt of their ire, and while we can't be expected to put up with abusive behavior, allowing families to vent can be a very useful intervention, even if it was never covered in Nursing 101."

We've usually found that families are grateful to be included and can be quite helpful with monitoring and reinforcement of the therapeutic things you've been teaching your patients. If anyone can get Mr. Pulasky to use his incentive spirometer, it will be his granddaughter or Mrs. Pulasky! We have also found that if a family member must be asked to vacate an area temporarily or other situations arise, giving an explanation and a time limit to the forced absence allows the family to be able to tolerate it more comfortably.

This leads to the touchy subject of having family present in a code situation. There are different schools of thought on this, but research and present-day practices are leaning more and more toward the beneficial aspects of allowing family to witness code activity. Generally, family get to see that everything possible was done for their loved one. No mystery or fear of inadequate care lingers. They get to say good-bye if a patient does die (and during the death, not after, which is an important aspect of the grieving process); and they can, if they legally have power of attorney, stop procedures to allow dignity in dying or decreased suffering. This is the ultimate act of family/patient advocacy, what each one of us would want if the situation were our own.

This leads us to the good ol' saying, "Do unto others as you would have done to you." Why is this such an easy thing to say and such a hard thing to practice?! We all have the same needs for respect and recognition of our humanity as do our patients and their families. We all have to try and remember this, even and especially when our nerves are frazzled and Ms. Green is climbing the side rails, Mr. Green is yelling at us, and it's 2 p.m. and we've only had two cups of coffee and a grabbed handful of Doritos to eat so far. Don't worry, you'll have plenty of time to practice your stellar, compassionate, empathetic people-skills in nursing!

Quality Peer Relations and Teamwork

Nursing is a stressful—albeit rewarding—job. One of the things (and possibly one of the most important) that can tip the scale way too close to the stress critical mass side, is difficult or adversarial peer relationships. Even though you will be working with nurses—similarly trained and with the same goals of competent patient care in mind, we are all still individuals—with our life and work experiences, personality types, and foibles intact.

Our peer relations can be an uplifting, inspirational joy, our greatest professional support, or a taxing misery. Alas, we cannot control the personalities of others. So the place to start looking at peer relationships is with ourselves, since our coworkers' behaviors will often be reactions to our own behavior.

To start, when you begin a new position, you should expect a period of time when your peers will be checking you out. What do we mean? For instance, your coworkers may ask you about previous jobs, the nursing school you went to, personal information, etc. You may notice that people are watching your medication administration technique, or how you handle a critical patient. Luckily, at least at this juncture, nurses are so sorely needed, that a new face on the unit is a welcome sight and so usually you will be greeted with delight (at least initially).

But invariably, there will be a nurse who must test the waters by challenging you in some way. This can be questioning something you're doing, speaking to you in a hostile, authoritarian, or condescending tone, or ignoring you completely. In the past, Staci had an experience when starting a new position in which she and one other nurse had to prepare meds for 30 people. This procedure took more than an hour overall and was accomplished in a narrow rectangular room, approximately 8 feet x 5 feet, with the doors locked shut (this was a psychiatric facility). The veteran nurse refused to utter one word to Staci throughout the entire procedure, deigning to even reach over her to obtain, let's say, the pill crusher, instead of asking her for it. She attempted to act as if Staci was completely nonexistent. This is an extreme example of challenging behavior, but some form of "testing" is normal. This "newbie" time must be looked at as opportunity time. You have the opportunity to set up how coworkers will perceive you. When faced with this situation, go out of your way to calmly introduce yourself to everyone in your area. Make a point to ask questions about the office's/unit's procedures. Ask specific nurses how they handle such and such situation. Use the ever-important eye contact.

During the "testing time" it's especially important to not be late and to not linger past your shift, and to make extra sure you follow the dress code to the letter. It might help if you consider the "newbie" time an extension of the interviewing process; now it's just your fellow employees sizing you up! If and when you are treated condescendingly or hostilely, etc., it's always important to step back from the situation before reacting. Remember this person is baiting you, so don't give him the satisfaction of taking the bait! It is also important to remember that this behavior (especially because he doesn't even know you yet) has to do with the offending person and his issues, not you. When possible, and a private moment is at hand, you will need to address the behavior directly.

We know you heard this before, but you just *have* to use "I" statements, such as "I was confused by your tone of voice when we spoke a few minutes ago. Being new, did I do something to offend you that I wasn't aware of?" or, related to condescension, "I appreciate the way you explained that procedure to me earlier, that was nice of you. It's always great when people go out of their way to be helpful and kind to the new person."

You may notice you're not attacking back, but you are asserting yourself as well as proving you are an up-front, problem-solving kind of human. The second scenario may sound a little sarcastic, but say it with a genuine demeanor. The offending peer will pick up your meaning, will recognize you're not going to take any guff, and will hopefully start to look at you as an equal. Up front, eye-to-eye discussion is always the way to handle this behavior.

One attitude that almost never wins friends and influences people is the "newbie know it all." Even if you do have lots of related experience, acting as if everything being done by this unit is wrong or inefficient, or going about spouting your credentials, etc., will not help you assimilate into the unit smoothly. Even if you have great ideas about quality control or the newest products, give yourself and your new place time to get used to each other. Change is stressful and downright scary to some. If your manager and peers get to know you and, importantly, trust you, they will welcome ideas for increased productivity and the like.

Feeling like you need to prove yourself is normal. Do it with actions and sincerity. Be there to help pull a patient up or to cover for a coworker so she can go to her kid's graduation. Do not fall into the trap that really springs from insecurity—boasting.

You may be wondering how Staci handled "the silent treatment" from the veteran nurse? Well, they were already alone (in the room). When the meds were all set up Staci began to chuckle and said, " I didn't know we had taken a vow of silence when we came to work here, that was the quietest med pour I've ever done!" She looked at the silent nurse directly, smiled, chuckled a little more, and left the room. The episode never reoccurred and, grudgingly at first but then wholeheartedly, this nurse came around and a pleasant, mutually valued professional relationship ensued.

So we know from experience you really can sweeten up curmudgeons, to the curmudgeon's and your benefit. Why bother? Because you will need allies in your practice. You will have bad days when you don't want to end up working with people you consider "enemies" and— guess who's on the schedule! And many times, these veterans have helpful information to impart that you could miss if all you do is snipe at each other. Again, remember this is about the person, not you. One can even check their impressions out with other peers—carefully (meaning, don't go to the next nurse you see and say, "What the heck is the matter with that miserable...") by asking, ("I" statements again) "I seemed to have upset Morticia just now," etc. You may hear that this is a pattern or the general modus operandi, therefore having even less to do with you.

Being able to calmly and nondefensively state your concerns, questions—and this relates to all people you will work with, such as administrators, nurses, doctors, managers—will always portray you as an intelligent professional worthy of respect. There are some particular incidences that are true conflicts and will require advanced conflict resolution skills. Please check out Conflict Resolution for some specific coping mechanisms for these small to large crises.

As you and your coworkers get used to each other and you have felt out the many different personality types, your personal style will become part of the style of the unit. It will be part of what, hopefully, will be a team approach. Although most facilities follow a primary care approach to patient care, you and your coworkers will need to utilize each other's strengths, muscles, and brain cells to give the highest quality patient care possible coupled with the lowest nursing stress level.

We're all taught to get help when transferring or lifting patients. We also need to utilize each other's skills when faced with an ethical dilemma, or a difficult med calculation, or when we're at the end of our

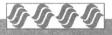

Conflict Resolution

First of all, request to see the person you are having the issue with in private and remember these simple guidelines:

- No public arguing.
- Use "I" statements only when addressing your concerns.
- Use eye contact.
- Be aware of the rules of body language. It is possible to sabotage open communication unconsciously by the way you hold your body in relation to the other person. For example, men usually do not stand closely face to face as it can be perceived as threatening. One person facing front and one person facing at an angle is a more relaxed positioning for discussion.
- Women are more comfortable with face-to-face interaction.
- Maintain open and sufficient personal space with everyone.
- Use the facts of the situation to corroborate your argument.
- Allow the person to make points without interruption.
- Demand (calmly) your right to the same non-interruption.
- Keep this type of meeting short; 15 minutes or so.

Second, if this leads only to an impasse, request a meeting with your supervisor present.

- Remember to always use the chain of command.
- Work toward resolution with an eye on workable compromise for both parties whenever possible. Winner/loser situations are almost always set-ups for future problems.
- Most facilities have mediation boards, ethics hot lines, etc., available when situations are beyond the scope or ability of immediate supervisory resolution. If the problem is an ethical issue and retaliation or other legal fears are a concern, it is feasible to go straight to the ethics hot-line route to report your concern. Many of these hot-lines complaints can be reported anonymously and strict confidentiality codes are utilized.

Conflict resolution related to patients

For violent, hostile or psychiatrically impaired patients:

- Attempt to use a calm voice, speaking quietly and using the most respectful use of the person's name/title as possible.
- Do not touch a patient that appears fearful or angry.
- Do not isolate yourself with an angry patient.
- Do not block a patient's escape route, or your own. Do not allow a patient to be between you and an exit.

(continued)

- Always make sure that your coworkers know the situation you are dealing with. If necessary, have staff and security at close range for assistance. This does not mean to crowd the patient with people or security, as this is a sure-fire way to escalate a problem.
- Do not attempt to argue with patients about their hallucinations, you will only engender escalated hostility and suspicion.
- Reiterate that you want to help patients feel safe. State that you are there to try to help them but you need their help to do this.
- State reality when necessary—who you are, why you want patients to comply with your requests, where they are, etc.
- If patients appear to be calming down, approach slowly and gauge their response as you do. Back off if necessary.
- If the situation seems to have relaxed enough that you are able to see patients recognizing you as a nonthreat and they are VERBALLY stating they understand what you want and what you are going to do (place an IV line, for example), make no moves without a brief verbal check first. For example, "Okay, Henry, are you ready? Just like we discussed. I'm going to try and get your IV now, it will be a quick needle stick now, are you ready?' Also make eye contact and smile. Remember to have an associate very close by to assist you if necessary.
- You will need to repeat multiple times what you want to do and why; it is helpful to ask the patient if they understand and attempt to smile at them, making eye contact at this time.
- From the beginning, always validate their discomfort. Verbalize that you see that they are upset and want to assist them.

In specific situations, a patient can react so rapidly that you may find yourself doing damage control instead of therapeutic interaction. A nurse should never enter a dangerous situation alone when possible. If a patient unexpectedly attacks you and there is assistance at hand, the damage can be kept then to a minimum. There are other situations in which a confused, psychotic, inebriated, etc., patient must be restrained for his or her own safety. Each facility has its own rules and regulations related to these procedures, and these should be carefully reviewed during your orientation. Some general points are:

- Four people are necessary to properly restrain a combative patient; one per limb.
- The approach is discussed before the attempt. The nurse in charge of the patient decides which staff member will maintain which limb. That person should focus on controlling that limb specifically (e.g., holding it down and placing the restraint).
- It is still important for ONE (the nurse in charge of the patient) person to try to quietly and briefly explain what is going on and why to the patient. Maintain as much dignity for the patient as possible.

(continued)

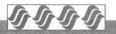
- Never tie restraints to moving parts of a stretcher, for example, side-rails, as you can injure a patient's arm or leg in doing so.
- A restrained patient needs to be kept visible to staff at all times (1:1).
- Follow, check, and ADL (bathroom, water, turning, etc.) guidelines carefully.
- Document carefully using your facility's specific restraint documentation paperwork.
- Restraints must occur only with a written doctor's order and renewed with another order as per your institution's guidelines.

Some other general points of self-protection are:

- If a patient bites you, do not wrench your arm, leg, etc., from her mouth. Press the affected body part deeper into her mouth, either holding it there to avoid increased ripping damage or forcing the patient to open her mouth because of the pressure, allowing you to extricate yourself.
- Hold a patient's hand to your head, with both hands if necessary, if your hair is being pulled. Pulling away may leave some of your scalp behind.
- If a patient grabs you around the neck with his arm, attempt to force your chin down between his arm and your throat to protect your airway. Attempt to turn your lowered chin toward the crook of his elbow if possible to increase breathing space.

There are many more self-defense tactics and strategies that can be useful to nurses. These are especially important for nurses who will be practicing in ERs, psychiatric facilities, etc. Your institution should provide inservices as well as literature related to these strategies.

We're not trying to scare you, just make you aware and begin to get you thinking. Experience will be a great teacher, but preparation and prevention, as well as good therapeutic technique can minimize negative experiences of this sort. Demand that your place of business educate you and ancillary staff (security, etc.) about how to handle conflict and violence.

rope and out of solutions pertaining to a difficult patient, and so on. You will quickly figure out who is the best IV stick on the floor, who handles the psychiatrically challenged patients best, and who is the finest at time management/organization dilemmas. Asking questions and working together has the somewhat counterintuitive effect of making you smarter and more efficient as well as the person who may have helped you. No one wants to feel alone in a difficult or strenuous situation. If possible, assist your coworkers with their patient care and be assertive enough to ask for the same in return. The care will go faster and smoother if you do so.

Cross-Generational Concerns

As professionals, older and younger nurses share many of the same goals. This common ground should be the starting point for professional relationships. Beyond that, the consensus among "seasoned" professionals seems to be that younger, less experienced nurses need to be open, nay, eager to learn. They need to ask questions, be open to suggestions, and need to recognize the value of experience. This and displaying professional behavior (taking your position seriously) will earn the respect of your veteran counterparts. The worst sins within a new nurse–old nurse situation (in the eyes of the veteran) is arrogance and defensiveness on the part of the greenhorn. As for the new nurse, compassion and an openness of mind are the prized qualities hoped for from an experienced nurse. New nurses, sometimes because they see old problems with fresh eyes, can and do have great ideas. Their boundless energy is a wonderful asset as well. It is yet another truth that respect must flow both ways in order to achieve an optimal working environment.

Dating in the Workplace

The nurses we surveyed gave wildly disparate (OK not really wildly, but definitely disparate) answers to questions about dating within the workplace. These answers ranged from, "Not only did I date someone where I worked, I married him; what a wonderful opportunity!" to "Dating someone where you work is one of the worst mistakes anyone can make."

There does not seem to be one perfect answer to this question, although certain specific situations lend themselves to clearer parameters. It is always considered unethical, and in some instances, grounds for termination (e.g., in the military) for staff employees to date supervisors, administrators, etc. Real issues related to favoritism, sexual harassment, nonprofessionalism, etc., abound with these situations, and will make a working environment less than favorable for you or your coworkers. Any time someone has a position of authority above your own, that power inequality is a set-up for issues within the relationship and suspicion among the people you work with. This is at its worst with immediate bosses, but applies to your institution in general as well. This also applies to patient-nurse dating. Of course, if a mutual attraction occurs with a patient, that can be pursued outside of the place of business. If a relationship with a supervisor seems inevitable, you or the supervisor will need to at least resign from the specific unit, etc., where his/her authority affects you and your coworkers. At times, the only solution is for you or your paramour to move to another facility altogether. Although this may seem dramatic, the drama and possible legal ramifications in the workplace would be far greater. As for nurses dating nurses at the same staff level, this seems to be generally accepted. Many concerns still arise when the two nurses are on the same unit, concerns that echo the ones above. It is still probably a good idea to keep romance at least one area removed, if possible. Easy to say but hard to do when love calls, eh? (Does anyone hear violin music?) If you must date within your own roster of nurses, it behooves both of you to be extra careful not to play favorites with each other, remember to assist your coworkers, and especially keep public interaction completely G-rated and professional! I know we don't have to mention no hanky-panky in the clean utility room, but also, keep the terms of endearment outside, no hand-holding, etc. It's also important to remember that even if sexual/romantic activity is not directed at a specific person, that person can validly and officially charge you with sexual harassment if made to feel uneasy enough by your behavior.

The other issue you should ponder is how will you handle the situation when, er, if the relationship goes sour. When the party's over but you have to keep "dancing" on the 3 to 11 shift with Mary, oy vey can that be difficult. Fighting, sniping, revenge of any kind is almost as bad as hanky-panky in the clean utility room. Running to the bathroom every 5 minutes to cry (because you have no room to resolve your feelings as your ex walks past you every 3 minutes) is not conducive to good time-management or sanity. You will not be able to ignore each other either. This will make your love-life a focus of the whole unit, which, of course, is not very pleasant. We have found that the space and intensity of nursing and the focus it demands can be a panacea and wonderful coping tool when dealing with painful matters of the heart. When your own personal heart pain is in your face at work every day, that coping mechanism is taken from you. Think carefully and wisely when pursuing relationships in the workplace and remember the general rule that if you work in the same institution with your main squeeze, the more space between both of you, the better.

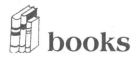 **books**

Eldgin, Suzette Haden (2000).
The Gentle Art of Verbal Self Defense. New York, NY: Prentice Hall Press.

This classic book, originally published in 1980, is now somewhat dated, but it does an excellent job of describing the many ways human beings attempt to manipulate one another. Also includes lots of practice exercises and practical tips.

Eldgin, Suzette Haden (1995).
You Can't Say That to Me: Stopping the Pain of Verbal Abuse. New York, NY: John Wiley and Sons.

This is a much more up-to-date book on verbal self-defense; it is particularly good for dealing with situations in which there is a great power imbalance between you and the person with whom you are setting verbal boundaries. The same author also has written books on verbal self-defense for parents and kids, and parents and teens.

Jeffers, Susan (1998).
Feel the Fear and Do It Anyway. New York, NY: Ballantine Books.

This book (which is also available on CD or as a download from www.audible.com) is about setting goals and going after them. The very best sections of the book, however, are about dealing with the people around you while working toward your goals; for example, how to get your significant other on board. The author includes actual case studies and role-playing exercises. The section on "no lose" decisions should be required reading for anyone undergoing a transition time in life.

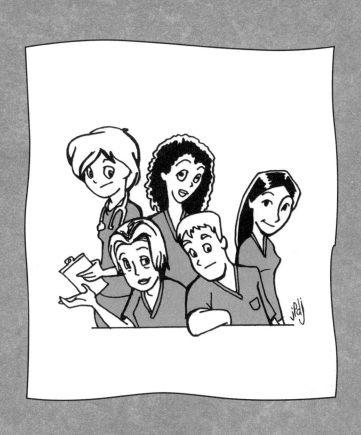

Diversity in Nursing

A Nurse Speaks

"I hear a lot about diversity, but I don't understand what it means. Can't we all just get along?"

TY, RN, New York state

 Importance of Diversity

T his chapter is about what it means, how it works, and how it can work better for members of minority groups within nursing. We've chosen to write about groups that have historically been either underrepresented in nursing or may encounter particular barriers because of their minority status. The groups we've chosen to include are nurses of color, men in nursing, lesbian, gay, bisexual and transgender nurses (we'll use the abbreviation LGBT from now on), nurses with physical and mental health–related disabilities, and nurses returning to the field.

Even if you don't identify with belonging to any particular minority group, you'll undoubtedly have both coworkers and patients who belong to these groups, so our hope is that this chapter will be useful to all nurses.

The admonition to "honor diversity" has become so well used that the phrase teeters dangerously close to cliché. Ask the average individual what "honoring diversity" is all about and you'll get a vague answer, perhaps because the idea is amazingly simple while the practice is exceedingly complex.

At the simplest level, "honoring diversity" means doing all the things you learned about in kindergarten, such as being kind and treating people as you would like to be treated.

When you bring it down to actual practice, i.e., how do I treat a coworker who seems very different from me, it becomes more complicated because of cultural assumptions, stereotyping, and lack of information. All this is made even more complicated by the fact that one is seldom aware of assumptions one is making (we guess that's why they're called assumptions). But there are a few basic behavioral tenets that can help guide you through many interactions with coworkers and patients that seem very different from you, no matter if the difference is age, gender, sexual orientation, etc.

The first tenet is: allow people around you to self-identify.

For example, the nurse who you think "looks Asian" may in fact be Korean-American but has lived in the United States all of her life and may speak only English...and maybe the Spanish she learned in school. A patient's family member who has started to take hormones to begin the process of transitioning from male to female may use the pronoun "he" or "she." A nurse who was born in Mexico but moved to the United States when she was 10 years old may identify as Mexican-American, Mexican, Latina, American, or none of these. She might speak Spanish at home or she might not, or she might not speak Spanish at all. A patient who is married but occasionally has sex with men might identify as bisexual, or he might never use that word to describe himself. The key is not to assume either anyone's identity (the way they see themselves) or perhaps more importantly, what that identity will mean about their abilities or behavior.

Although we can sometimes feel ourselves stretching to understand a coworker or patient who might be different from us, it's important to recognize that the discomfort of this stretching is a positive thing. Honoring diversity is more than just not discriminating; it's about making sure that the gifts and energies of all individuals are honored. This ultimately (pardon us for sounding so "we are the world" about this) makes any workplace a better workplace.

Before we go on to the real substance of this chapter, we wanted to add that we realize that it is the nurses who are dealing with specific diversity issues (i.e., nurses of color, male nurses, etc.) who are the experts on these issues, and we've included their comments as much as possible. However, we appreciate the limitations of covering complex issues in such a short number of pages and we urge those with more interest and concern to investigate some of the many excellent resources we've referenced at the end of this chapter.

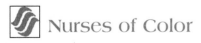 ## Nurses of Color

The term "person of color" has developed in the past decade and a half to describe individuals who identify as anything other than non-

Hispanic white (i.e., Caucasian). We're using the blanket term "nurses of color" not because all the groups it encompasses are the same but because some of the difficulties encountered are similar enough to warrant a collective discussion.

Some of the nurses we talked with who identify as "of color," stated that the most difficult time in their nursing career was their first nursing job. "I'd done all my clinical rotations in large urban hospitals near the nursing school I attended where the staff, nursing students and patients were a pretty heterogeneous group of all different races," said one female new grad who is African-American, "when I started applying to hospitals in the suburban area where my parents live, I began to get some funny reactions. No one said anything outright discriminatory—I guess people are too PC for that—but one nurse recruiter assumed I'd grown up in an urban area and another asked a 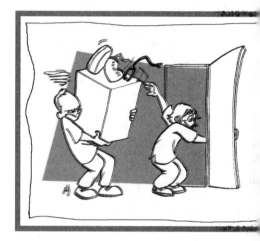 slightly clueless question about my hair. Both were just making casual conversation, but it was significant to me. I definitely could tell they hadn't been around African-American people much."

Other nurses agreed that although they had certainly experienced outright discrimination, most of the difficulty encountered from both staff and patients arose out of inexperience with people of color.

Janet Lincoln, an African-American ER nurse in California explains, "Sometimes it becomes clear in a conversation…halfway through I think, hmmm, you don't have any black friends do you? You can tell when you're talking to someone with a everything-I-need-to-know-about-black-people-I-learned-by-watching-the-WB attitude, they're always expecting stand-up comedy from me, which frankly makes me get very serious, very quick."

Certainly this (as Janet Lincoln says) "Everything I Need to Know About Black People I Learned by Watching the WB" attitude can have negative consequences for both staff members and patients. Some nurses nevertheless had strong hope that if nurses of different races and ethnicities were able to work together, it could lead to further understanding. "Dr. King said that Sunday morning [at church] was the most segregated time of the week, and that's still true in many areas," one hospice nurse from Ohio, who identifies as African-American, told us. "At the same time, the work day is often the least segregated time of the week. Go into almost any restaurant, even in large urban areas. If you see a group of all different races of people eating together, I can almost guarantee they're coworkers." This nurse went on to explain, "This can lead to real friendships, and friendships can help with understanding."

When asked what other types of things white nurses can do to have better relations with their non-white coworkers, the first reaction of most of the nurses we talked with was—don't be afraid to talk about differences.

"I'm not saying cross-examine me about Korean culture or pester me to teach you how to make kimchee from scratch," said one Korean-American RN who lives in Atlanta, "but it's okay to ask about [how] I celebrate holidays, just like you would with any other coworker."

"Don't always make the person of color mention race, especially if you think there might be a cultural difference going on," said one nurse who identifies as African-American. "I was in a staff meeting recently when there was a conflict of opinion, basically about a communication issue, and the staff was evenly divided about the issue right along racial lines. When one of the white nurses pointed this out and added 'hmmm I'm wondering if there are cultural issues we should examine' everyone let out the biggest collective sigh of relief you've ever heard from a group of people. After some more discussion we were able to come up with a reasonable compromise."

Another nurse mentioned that nurses of all colors should avoid what she calls "Bending over Blackwards." She related the following story: "Last year we had an incident at the hospital where I work. Over a few weeks a man had been groping women in the reception area. When one of the nurses wrote a warning on the dry-erase board she gave a physical description which included the words 'African-American gentleman.' Let's think about this; if he's groping women, is he actually a gentleman? Not by my definition, but I'm sure the nurse was trying to avoid describing him in a negative light related to race. But you don't have to offset the "African-American" with 'gentleman' because especially in this kind of situation it isn't a negative thing to include someone's race when you are giving a physical description of them."

Finally, one nurse mentioned that it's important to differentiate between different cultures and subcultures within cultures as well as beware of linguistic differences. "When I worked at one long-term care facility, the other nurses called all the clients who spoke Spanish 'Mexican" even though many of them were Dominican," said one nurse who is originally from Puerto Rico and now lives in Pennsylvania. "Okay, so we all speak Spanish, but that doesn't mean we necessarily have anything more in common culturally than that."

Men in Nursing

Although the percentage of nurses who are men has been rising for the past decade, the percentage of nurses who are men is still very small. People who are nurses—and guys—often say this is due to lack of male nurse role models.

"There's all sorts of stereotypes," said Craig Fellow, a dialysis nurse who lives in Alabama. "Male nurses are, let's see gay and/or got kicked out of medical school. Once, someone combined both stereotypes and asked me if I got kicked out of medical school for being gay. I had to resist an urge to say 'oh my God, yeah, how did you guess?' "

Even if amusing, such stereotypes undoubtedly prevent many men from even considering a career in nursing and can also contribute to problems on the floor.

"It's better now than before, but I still see it all the time," said Ed Bressler, who has been an ICU nurse for 15 years, "male new grads especially are so eager to prove they're 'all man' they do things like act super macho, lifting people they shouldn't be lifting without help, etc. This can—and often does—lead to injuries."

Mr. Bressler's statements lead nicely into the subject of what one nursing student called "Mr. Brawny Syndrome," or men doing an unfair amount of lifting or other physical work on the floors.

One male nurse described it this way, "For a while it was almost like a guarantee; if there was someone violent on the floor, they were going to be part of my assignment. But after my sixth shift in a row of taking care of all psychotic, morbidly obese s/p CVA folks, I need something a little different. I want to occasionally care for the little old lady on a morphine drip who just needs to talk. And it's probably important for her on some level too."

Male nurses agreed there is no one perfect way to deal with this problem, although most were able to speak directly with staff members who are the worst offenders. "It seems like each shift I have to deal with one staff person who always treats me as a lift-o-matic," says one male nurse, "and I do want to help out when I can, but there are limits. Any nurse who is always doing heavy lifting all the time, every shift every day, will develop a back injury over time. So I try and be direct without being difficult. I told one nurse who used to call me for help with every patient that I could only help her with three patients a shift because y'know, I have my own patient load. That way she knew I was available to help with the three most difficult situations but couldn't be available at her beck and call. She had to prioritize her need for my assistance."

Other proposed solutions to "Mr. Brawny Syndrome" include: talking to supervisors about the situation, advocating for a 'lifting team' with specialized training and equipment to be used in the most difficult situations, and faking a back injury (we're saying these solutions were proposed, not that we're particularly recommending all of them).

Another common difficulty mentioned by male nurses is what to do when addressed as "doctor." Some nurses said they corrected this perception each time, every day, but other nurses said they simply gave up.

"I introduce myself as 'your nurse' when I go into the room," said one nurse who has worked on a med/surg floor "since the dinosaurs roamed the earth." "It's obnoxious to keep saying nurse, nurse, nurse, nurse in response to doc, doc, doc, doc. Forget it. I know I'm a nurse and I tell the patient once each shift. That's all I can do. I know who I am."

Nurses with Physical and Mental Health–Related Disabilities

In recent years, the talents and employability of nurses with disabilities have become higher profile, featured in such regional nursing employment journals as *Nursing Spectrum* and *Advance for Nurses* and publicized through the Website ExceptionalNurse.com.

For nurses with a disability, the exposure is positive, but the unfortunate reality remains that the employment rate for all individuals with disabilities (including nurses) is still abysmally low.

To quote every stand-up comic who ever, well, stood up, "What's that about?"

It's about assumptions mostly; the assumption that a nurse with a disability won't be able to do the job. And while it's true that nurses with certain types of disabilities would not be able to perform the "essential functions" for certain types of nursing jobs, in other instances, with certain reasonable accommodations a nurse may very well be able to do another type of nursing job.

The key, say experts, is finding the fit between a nurse and a job, which may require some work and some openmindedness on the part of the nurse and the employer.

"As nurses, we all have strengths and weaknesses," said one nurse who is hard of hearing and works on a med/surg floor with the use of a vibrating pager that alerts her to call bells and an amplified stethoscope. "My weakness is my hearing, so if I feel unsure about breath sounds, I'll ask a coworker to double-check a patient for me. On the other hand, one of my strengths is my organizational abilities, so the new grads often come to me with questions about how to make the most of their time.

Often the idea of that a nurse is—dramatic pause—'hard of hearing' makes a situation seem high stakes for those who haven't been around an individual with a disability, but in reality it's a simple matter of working with each other's strengths and assisting others where they might need a hand."

This same nurse notes that recent technological advances (amplified stethoscopes, vibrating pagers) has improved employment possibilities for nurses who have sensory impairments, so more nurses are becoming familiar with the experience of working with a nurse with a disability. "It's really common sense," she says. "Don't assume things. I can't tell you how many people have seen my hearing aids and decided I must have trouble seeing too. I don't know, maybe they heard too many Helen Keller jokes as a child. But it just doesn't make sense. It makes me shudder a little to think, if nurses are assuming things like this about another nurse with a disability, what must they assume about their disabled patients?" To provide some enlightening—if satirical—instructions about interacting with an individual who has a disability, we've included *Taking the "Dis" Out of Disabled,* written by Maura Kelly, a disability rights advocate who often speaks to health-care providers about issues of disability and access to health care.

"It's important for nurses with any type of disability to stick together

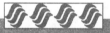

Taking the "Dis" Out of "Disabled"

By Maura Kelly

Maybe you've heard those radio public service announcements, explaining exactly how to speak, act, dress, and smell around all people with any type, form, or hint of disability. Unfortunately, for our brothers/sisters with disabilities, these ads simply do not go far enough in establishing the fact that all people with disabilities are exactly the same.

So, as a public service, disability rights advocate Maura Kelly presents her Handy-Dandy Foolproof, 100% Guaranteed Or Three Times Your Money Back Tips for Dealing with the People Formerly Known as "Jerry's Kids."

Tip #1

People with disabilities seldom leave their beds, let alone their homes. Whenever you see disabled people on the street, know that just being out is a huge victory and a great and glorious occasion for them. Always stop to congratulate them on their inspirational foray into the real world. This is true even if they seem to be in a hurry. After all, they have a disability, where could they have to go?

(continued)

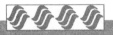
Tip #2
Remember, a person with a disability in one area is compensated by nature by having superhuman powers in another area. For example, all visually impaired people have exceptional hearing and all hearing-impaired people can read lips from a mile or more away.

Tip #3
If a person with a disability smiles or winks at you from across the bar, be assured he is not flirting, but trying to ask you for your assistance in helping to go to the restroom. Physically assist the person to the bathroom stall immediately. Ignore all protests.

Tip #4
If a person with a disability seems to need help, or asks you for help in negotiating an architectural barrier, remember the person could not have *possibly* dealt with this situation previously and will therefore have no valuable input in what to do. Just do whatever you think will work, and ignore irrelevant verbal instructions on their part.

Tip #5
You are remembering this is satire, right?

Tip #6
When encountering persons with a disability for the first time, if they are accompanied by a seemingly able-bodied individual, assume that this person is their personal care attendant. Additionally, always direct communication through the personal care attendant. Talking directly to persons with a disability will only confuse them.

Tip #7
When you have social contact with a couple that includes one individual who has a disability, be extremely generous in your praise of the able-bodied partner. Sprinkle the words "sacrifice," "selfless," and "sisterhood" liberally throughout the conversation.

Tips #8 (and most important of all)
All people with disabilities are inspirational. Even though every day for them is torture, they still manage to put on a happy face to make able-bodied people feel more comfortable. So give the lil' troupers a gentle pat on the head, or slip them a dime in their fast food drink cup (they didn't want to finish that Diet Coke anyway). It's the least you can do.

Tip # 9
Hey, you did remember this is satire, right?

and to know our rights," says one nurse who has been hospitalized with clinical depression. "The first issue that is always brought up in the hiring process of a nurse with a disability is 'well now we have to think of the safety of our patients.' This is perfectly reasonable and, of course, the most important consideration when any nurse—disabled or not—is caring for patients. But sometimes it's even the tone of voice that makes it difficult. The implication is that, of course, I haven't thought of the safety of the patients. I think it speaks more to the interviewer's discomfort with a person with a disability than the actual way we can—or can't—make the situation work."

This discomfort with disability can be particularly exacerbated for nurses who became disabled from an on-the-job injury. Some nurses reported that even if they were able to be accommodated by the floor, other RNs, especially those they knew before the injury, treated them differently. LJ, a 10-year veteran who requested that her whole name not be used, recently returned to work after being out 9 months with what could have been a career-ending back injury.

"No one knew what to say," she remembers. "Nurses just don't want to think about not being able to function. It's part of the "nurses' personality" that we act as if we are invincible. Many of us eat junk all the time, smoke like fiends, don't get any exercise (running for call lights is a good start but probably not enough), and don't ask for help when lifting. We don't want to think anything we can't overcome is going to happen to us. So when the other nurses on the floor had to deal with someone who did have a severe work related injury, even though I'm 70% recovered, it freaked them out a bit. The saying goes, 'disabled' is the only minority group that any person, given the right circumstances of an accident, illness etc., can instantly be a part of. It's scary to think about, but it should give us all reason to pause and consider how to best use the talents of someone whose body doesn't work just like ours."

Lesbian, Gay, Bisexual, and Transgender Nurses

Many of the nurses we talked with who identify as lesbian, bisexual, gay or transgendered reported experiencing difficulty in being "out of the closet" (i.e., open about one's sexual orientation or in some cases, the complexity of one's gender identity).

"No one at work knows I'm gay and that's the way I like it," explained a home health nurse working in Wisconsin, "I've been out in other job situations and been completely hassled. One job, I came in to find the words 'ugly dyke' scrawled across my locker in indelible ink. It's a small place...someone had to have seen the person do it. But no one admitted it and the management—despite my request—never did a thing to address it, even indirectly."

"I refuse to be 'in the closet,' " said an ER nurse from Ontario, Canada, "When I first started my career I worked at a Catholic hospital so I felt like I had to be closeted and it was torturous. When my partner of 15 years died, I couldn't explain the situation to anyone, and I had to go in the next shift and act as if nothing had happened. I decided from that moment on that in honor of my partner—and out of respect for my own mental health—I would never ever ever be secretive about who I love again. I don't have to rent a billboard or wear a tee shirt that says 'guess what I'm gay' to be honest about who I am, but I'm not changing pronouns anymore either."

A more difficult issue even than the question of being out to coworkers is the issue of how to respond to patients who inquire—either out of curiosity or other motivations—about a nurse's sexual orientation.

"Giving care is always about the patient, it's never about the nurse," said a Texas RN who identifies as a lesbian, "but at the same time, sometimes patients will ask directly and I always say, 'Well why is it important for you to know because that's a somewhat personal question.' Sometimes they're just curious, other times the patient is gay and is struggling in some way. And of course, occasionally the patient asks because they don't want to be taken care of by a gay person."

Other LGBT nurses report similar situations. "I have asked for a changed assignment if a patient seems extremely homophobic or has made comments to other staff," said a gay male nurse from New York. "My nurse manager has always been understanding of my desire not to be the target of anyone's ire for an entire shift, and at the same time has never pressured me to change to confirm a patient's prejudice."

Some LGBT nurses reported frustrations because coworkers saw their identity as "all about sex," while the nurses themselves see having a lesbian, gay, bisexual, or transgendered identity as much more all encompassing.

In addition, some nurses found that their coworkers seeing them as only sexual and therefore "supersexual" was both offensive and limiting, a kind of objectification for entertainment value.

"I do have coworkers who assume I am Mr. Hyper Sexual," said one gay male nurse. "And it can be a pain when that's all someone can see me as. When we go on break together, there's this one nurse who always wants to hear about my adventures. Well, I have occasional adventures, like most single people, but she has an extremely exaggerated idea of my love life. I feel like saying 'it's not just gay people that have sex. *Sex in the City* is actually about straight women, right?' "

A number of nurses—regardless of their sexual orientation—talked about the experience of being seen as gay, usually because the nurse's appearance or mannerisms didn't match those traditionally associated with their gender (e.g., a woman with very short hair). In the case of a number of male nurses we talked with, simply being a nurse was enough to make people assume they were gay (or, of course, a doctor).

This brings us to the difficulty that the cultural norm of supporting a rigid gender binary brings to the nursing world and (pardon our intensity here) the world in general.

When we talk about this rigid gender binary we mean the way culture tells us what "real men" and "real women" act or look like. It's undoubtedly one of the reasons so few men go into nursing; surely a "real man" would not be interested in a "nurturing" profession, since nurturing is seen as a traditionally female trait. Yet there are many men who have nurturing personalities and there are many women who don't.

This leaves some male nurses in the difficult position of feeling they need to defend their masculinity. As one male oncology nurse said, "I admit it, my first year as a nurse I spent the whole time going 'my girlfriend this, my girlfriend that' just so everyone would know I wasn't gay; I guess I was defending my manhood. Finally one of my coworkers said 'dude no one cares if you're gay or straight or both or neither or whatever. You notice if someone's IV is infiltrating and that's what we care about around here."

 ## Nurses Returning to the Workforce

Nurses leave nursing for many reasons; burnout, to take care of children or aging parents (or not uncommonly, both), boredom, fatigue, tired of going home covered in other people's body fluids, etc. The body fluid issue notwithstanding, nurses usually return to the field because the reasons they left are either no longer an issue or the draw of nursing itself becomes stronger than the forces that drove the nurse out.

If you're an RN thinking of returning to the field, we have one thing to say to you (c'mon everyone join us)—Welcome! The nursing shortage isn't going away anytime soon, so those of us running around hospital floors, nursing homes, etc., like proverbial headless chickens are very glad for the help. And okay, it's not going to be easy (nothing much is easy in life, with the exception of sitting on the couch watching TV), but we're glad you're thinking of coming back to us.

We know you've thought long and hard about this decision. Nonetheless, before you totally commit yourself to this process, we suggest you take out a piece of paper (go on, you can even rip the last page out of this book if it's blank on one side) and draw a line down the middle. To the left of the line write "I left nursing because..." and begin to list the reasons. Try not to censure yourself, just keep writing. There may be more reasons (or fewer reasons) than you had originally thought. When you're done with your list put it aside for a while, go get a choco-mocha-frap-a-latte at your local independently owned coffee shop, read a paperback novel that will keep you completely absorbed (something by Stephen King might work perfectly), and then after a while look back over your paper. With the benefit of a bit of time, you may find that you've forgotten some reasons, or that what you called a "reason" was not a motivating factor at all. If it has been more than a few years since you worked as a nurse, you might also talk to someone who you were close to when you made the decision to leave nursing. The venting of a friend unhappy at work seems to be something humans remember a long time; perhaps it's some kind of evolutionary coping mechanism. At any rate, you can use this to your advantage by cross-examining the people who love you (and who knew you back in the day) about why they think you left nursing.

Of course, if you left, for example, to have children, the answer may be pretty straightforward (and your spouse might think it a wee bit odd that you're even asking) but double-check anyway. Speaking of kids, if you can find a somewhat sneaky way of getting them to talk about it (well, actually, you could ask directly) your kids might be able to give you interesting—and probably scathingly honest—information about their impression of how you liked your life as a nurse. If you came home always crabby, consistently complained about a particular supervisor, or never seemed rested when you worked third shift, they may well remember it and won't sugarcoat this info for you. Conversely, if they remember how you talked about patients or often glowingly shared how you had made a difference at work, or seemed more contented (if more tired) at the end of a day in your nursing life, they'll probably share that with you, too.

Once you have your reasons for leaving worked out, turn your attention to the other side of the paper, and write the reasons you want to go back, specifically addressing each reason you left. To use a no-brainer example, if you left nursing because you developed a bad back and you've since had physical therapy, done exercises, seen a faith healer, etc., and your back is fine, you can write "bad back" on one side and "back got better" on the other.

After another little break (maybe go for another choco-mocha-frap-a-latte), sleep on it (okay, we should have said a decaf choco-mocha-frap-a-latte) and the next morning look at your list with fresh eyes. Do the reasons for returning outweigh the reasons for leaving? Is there any area in which you need more information, or are you ready to make a decision?

Please, note we are not trying to discourage you with this little exercise (heck, we want you to come work at our jobs so we'll have another set of capable RN hands). However, in talking with returning nurses (some who were not completely thrilled with their decisions 6 months or so into it), we were occasionally reminded that despite the fact that most career handbooks talk of nursing as a calling, a number of nurses become nurses as a survival tactic. For example, perhaps they were in a hole financially, or seeking the wherewithal to get out of an abusive relationship (more than one nurse educator we talked with mentioned the high percentage of their female students who left situations of domestic violence immediately after getting their first job), or they're the first individual in their family to attend college and nursing seems the option most accessible to them, etc. There's nothing wrong with this choice; if a person has the aptitude and a reasonable amount of compassion, becoming a nurse because one has certain survival needs is not only reasonable and acceptable, it's brilliant. Actually, if in one's state of desperation, the idea of becoming a nurse seemed reasonable enough to someone, then they're obviously the kind of person who should become a nurse; the "caring about other humans" requirement is clearly met or their first inclination would have been toward being a diesel mechanic or something similar. By the end of nursing school, most have had the experience of ducking so as not to be hit with projectile vomit, and we still finished school. How much more evidence of suitability is needed? One does not need a "calling" to be an RN; we're nurses, not nuns.

Yes, dear reader, we can hear you thinking, "Thanks for the philosophical treatise on motivational possibilities for individuals attending nursing school, but would you mind explaining how all this relates to those considering returning to the nursing field?" We're so glad you asked! You see, if you became a nurse to meet some basic survival needs (e.g., safety, financial security) and you're in a place in your life where those needs can be met in other ways, you may find you're no longer able to tolerate some of the very real difficulties of life as a nurse. And this is a good thing; it means you've moved up further on Maslow's hierarchy of needs! But does this mean you shouldn't return to nursing? Not at all. It only means that you should think carefully about the things that were most difficult about the first part of your nursing career and try to avoid those things in part two.

Perhaps an illustration from the world of show business might be appropriate here. You've probably heard the story about singing superstar Patti LaBelle's nightly supper, before she signed her first record deal.

Urban legend has it that she would buy an eight pack of hot dogs every week and each night she would eat a single hot dog for her evening meal. As the story goes, she didn't have money to get her gas turned on, however, so each night she cooked her hotdog over the 100-watt light bulb in her shadeless lamp. Miss LaBelle is doing quite well now, and although we aren't personal friends with her, we can imagine that if she gets a hankerin' for a hot dog, she's not looking around for a 100-watt light bulb to cook it over.

The same thing goes for you. When you graduated from nursing school, you may have worked night shift in a state prison that was a 45-minute drive away from your house, and even though you hated driving and hated night shift, you did it because you felt like you had to. If you are in a position where don't need to work as a nurse to survive, you wouldn't last if you tried to return to your new-grad position. However, thanks to your new nonsurvival state and the nursing shortage, you probably will not have to take a job you hate just to work as a nurse. The key here is to look at what (if anything) made you miserable and avoid it if you can.

This may sound simple and, of course, it's a common sense kind of issue, but it might take some teasing to figure out what you did and didn't like in your nursing jobs of yore. It might have been that you didn't like working night shift, or it might have been that you didn't like working the night shift when your children were young and now that they're teenagers you might prefer to be at home winding down when they're leaving for school so you can make sure they're on time to first period. Being realistic about the specific issues that were most difficult at your last job can help you find a new nursing job more suitable for you. If you loved the responsibilities of an RN at a long-term facility but didn't particularly care for working with older adults, perhaps there is a long-term care facility near you that caters to the needs of adults with disabilities, which would probably involve working with younger clients.

Of course, while you were living your life and undoubtedly going through many changes, nursing has been changing, too. What will be different now? The answer depends on when you left nursing, although most nurses we talked with said the two biggest changes were use of technology, and an increase in patient acuity.

Some of the increases in technology are welcome additions. "IV pumps make all the difference in the world," said Sheila Benson, who spent 15 years away from the bedside. "Okay the beeping for no good reason will drive you crazy, but it sure beats counting drops." Other differences mentioned by returning nurses included use of computers for charting (mostly with med administration, "Whatever happened to Kardex?" asked one nurse), many new meds and new ways of administering them, and an increase in supervisory responsibilities secondary to the use of assistive personnel in acute care facilities.

For a low-key, gradual reentry, you can start to reexpose yourself to the world of nursing either online through reading message boards or participating in nursing listservs (we've includes some sites to start out with in, where else, the Resources section) or by reading nursing journals. This will acquaint you with some of the changes in nursing technology as well as nursing culture. If you find that one particular listserv or site seems to be filled with arguments and/or complaining, don't assume this is representative of the current state of nursing as a whole. Folks just need a place to release some of the pent up frustrations of nursing life, and posting a vent on a message board is much safer and kinder than taking it out on coworkers and the family dog. Usually on the busier message boards sponsored by commercial sites, needless flame wars and spam-like posts are removed, which creates a more productive and pleasant message board perusing experience for you.

Even though many things about nursing and the RN role have changed, one thing hasn't—the patient still needs a compassionate, caring nurse. As returning RN Barbara Lemon told us, "It's all different now and at the same time, the fact that a patient needs us means it's all very much the same."

Getting Started

So, you've done some thinking, even (cliché warning) soul searching, and decided this is the time for you go back to working as a nurse. What's the first step?

If you've let your license lapse, run don't walk (or maybe skip, if you're really happy about your decision) to the Website for your state board of nursing. You can follow the link from the National Council of State Boards of Nursing's Website (http://www.ncsbn.org/). Once there, you can find the requirements for what's called license reinstatement. Requirements for license reinstatement vary quite widely from state to state, and can involve a lot of (what else?) paperwork, so you'll want to get started immediately (if not sooner).

If your license is still active, then you'll want to avail yourself of one of the increasingly popular refresher courses available through community colleges, health care facilities, and independent adult learning facilities.

There are many different refresher courses and types of refresher courses available right now, and deciding on the one that's best for you and your situation may be somewhat challenging. To help you with your decision, check out the tips found in Choosing a Refresher Course.

Choosing a Refresher Course

The first consideration for choosing a refresher course is, does the course have a clinical component? Every nurse we talked with, from new grads working with returning nurses to nurse recruiters to returning nurses themselves said that if it doesn't have a clinical component, forget it.

One nurse who took a book and classroom-only class explained, "It just made me more nervous…and I didn't think that was possible. All day we'd hear about all these things that have changed since the 'olden days' but we never had a chance to try anything for ourselves. I was having nightmares until I quit and changed to a class that had a lab and an on-the-floor experience. I lost money but I didn't care. Changing was worth it."

Other considerations include:

How long is the class? How much time is devoted to classroom learning and how much of the time is clinical?

What is the average class size?

Who are the instructors? Are they familiar with adult learners? Are they currently practicing as nurses? Is this different for the clinical versus classroom instructors?

What are the costs involved? In addition to tuition, are there other fees or equipment that need to be paid for out of pocket?

What percentage of nurses complete the course and what percent go on to bedside nursing?

What are the prerequisites for starting the course? For example what paperwork do you need to have filled out? Do you need basic CPR? CPR for the health-care provider?

How long is the course? Is there any flexibility in scheduling, for example, does the facility offer a weekends only course, online options, etc.

If a student feels like they need additional practice or instruction, how do they get extra help? Is the skills lab open for practice? Is faculty help available? Are there instructional aides like videos and CDROMs students can take home?

How are students in the refresher course evaluated? Will there be written tests, return demonstrations, etc. If a student needs more help or more time for a specific aspect of the course or to refresh a certain skill, what provisions are made for this?

What kind of clinical supervision is provided?

Can you talk to someone else who took the course?

Finding a Job and Making It Work

Once you've started your refresher course, your thinking will naturally begin to focus on the next step, where will you work? Many refresher programs offer job placement or have a cooperative arrangement in place where they reimburse the cost of the course if you work for their facility for a set amount of time. Even if these possibilities are open to you, you may want to think about planning a job search of sorts, if even just to keep your options open.

If you've already read Chapter 2, you know everything there is to know (well, okay, everything we know) about writing a nursing resume, but of course you'll want to consider using the functional format to emphasize your skills rather than your recent nursing experience (or lack thereof). Be prepared, of course, to explain your long gaps in nursing employment (if you've not worked as a nurse for 15 years, it will be clear on even the slickest of functional resumes) but also be prepared to share why you're getting back into the field. If you review your handy "I left because..." worksheet from earlier in the chapter before the interview, you'll be exquisitely ready for this question. Especially highlight your success in the clinical components of the refresher course, which tells the recruiter that you're really ready for the challenges of nursing today.

As we mentioned in Chapter 2, don't let fear narrow or prematurely rule out any area of nursing for you. Many returning nurses have jumped right into the ICU or other technology intensive environments. "The local urban hospital offered an intensive care unit refresher program where I knew I would get the teaching and the help that I needed. I also thought that if I went into an environment with less machines, I would always be technology phobic. I guess I would say it was sink or swim but I never felt sinking was an option because of all the training and my long preceptorship. I figured that I had a very capable life vest and as long as I kept paddling I'd be just fine," said Carrie Atkins, a metaphorically inclined nurse currently practicing in Nevada.

Finally, join a support group and/or find a mentor. The support group doesn't have to be anything fancy, or even formal. The group could easily be made up of some fellow students from your refresher course, an old nursing school buddy who also recently returned to the floor (who says two people isn't a group?), or even an acquaintance you make online through one of the nursing discussion boards or general nursing listservs. At the time this book was written, we scoured the net looking for listservs specifically for returning nurses but couldn't find any. Maybe you should surf over to one of the free group hosting services (www.yahoogroups.com comes to mind) and start one of your own!

The Graying of the RN Workforce

The "graying of the RN workforce" is the somewhat euphemistic phrase that describes the fact that the average age of an RN is increasing. It is this fact, plus the belief that nurses must (or at least will) retire at a certain age, that leads to the most alarming projections about the nursing shortage.

If hospitals could find a way to encourage nurses to postpone the retirement of these valuable, experienced nurses (in a kinder way, hopefully than a nasty Enron-esque retirement earnings loss debacle), it would delay, at least, the height of the nursing shortage.

Some steps hospitals could take to make bedside nursing sustainable for the older nurse could be as simple as scheduling flexibility. Said one older nurse, "I can't do 12 hour shifts anymore. My feet ache too much and I don't have the stamina that I used to have. I'm still a good nurse, I've been awarded employee of the month twice in the last year, and I not only get my work done, but help out the younger gals and other new nurses when I'm finished. I wanted to go to 8-hour shifts and my nurse manager agreed, but this was vetoed at the next level. So they lost a good nurse because I went to a competing hospital that welcomed me to work 8-hour shifts."

Another tactic hospitals have used to decrease the physical stress of the job is to institute "lifting teams." While some nurses—of all ages—found this helpful, most emphasized that it's often the lifts that have to be done without the benefit of the specially trained team that are most risky to the backs of the nurses. For example, "If you have a patient on the floor in the shower, that's an extremely difficult lift," explained one nurse, "but if the patient is freezing and scared but otherwise okay you don't want to wait for the lift team. You want them back in bed, as cozy as possible, as soon as possible for both the patient's sake and in terms of liability." Other nurses are distrustful of interventions, such as lift teams, because they feel it's a slippery slope to nurses being even less involved in patient care.

Even if hospitals take the lead, most older nurses say, younger RNs also could use some understanding of the concerns and potential of older nurses. "We have nurses in their early twenties and nurses in their late fifties working here," said Janice Preston, who works in a long-term care facility in Chicago, Illinois. "When our youngest nurse and our oldest nurse are on at the same time, that's an almost 30-year difference in ages—between two people who are doing exactly the same job. You don't see that in many other professions. It can make for some interesting situations. A conversation about where you were when Kennedy got shot can be interrupted by one of the younger nurses saying 'Wow! That was 15 years before I was born!' It really brings home the difference when it's put in historical perspective like that. I never feel hurt or slighted by that kind of conversation because at least it's out in the open; I'm older than you by a lot of years, okay let's go on. It's the subtle things that make me feel my contribution isn't valued. Things like the younger nurses not asking me to go out with them after work, even if they're talking about their plans right in front of me. Or having a nurse assume I don't know about some new piece of technology. You think just because it has shiny buttons I won't be able to use it? Come on, I work right alongside you every day. Can't you see anything besides the gray hair?"

How can older nurses best deal with the insidious ageism that might make a younger nurse assume that an older nurse is less competent? Some nurses mentioned emphasizing one's physical fitness ("I take a Pilates class and a karate class and don't think I don't talk about it at work all the time"), being aware of "we-always-did-it-this-way-so-this-way-is-better" attitudes, and embracing the very technology older workers are assumed to fear. "Take a computer class!" said one nurse, who at 56 says she still has "a couple of more years of floor nursing in this ol' body." She goes to explain, "Last place I worked they started up with computer charting and the younger nurses took to it right away and the older nurses complained, complained, complained. I complained too, until I was tired of hearing myself. All this denigration of progress made me feel older than I was and I noticed a subtle shift in the way the younger nurses treated me too. They always used to ask me for help with lifting, etc., and I realized they had stopped. That made me feel so old. I knew I can lift a patient even if I can't use a mouse, but they didn't understand that. So before I went to my next job, I took a computer class at the community college where my nephew teaches. It was really helpful and now I feel comfortable with whatever they decide to put on the computer. I know some of the nurses call me 'techno-grandma' behind my back, but they don't treat me like an old lady and that's all I care about."

Among the over-50 set we talked with, most reiterated that they wanted to decide for themselves when they'd had enough. "I'm old, I don't mind admitting that," said a 52-year-old RN who currently works in Rochester, N.Y., "and nursing is a physically demanding job. To pretend that both those facts are not true is just silliness. The question is, can I do the work? Right now, I can, but a 50 year old back is not the same as a 25 year old back and I don't know how much longer I can be at the bedside. But I want it to be up to me to decide. I don't want to feel pushed out."

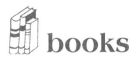 **books**

Boles, Richard Nelson (2000).
Job Hunting for the So-Called Handicapped or People Who Have Disabilities. Berkeley, CA: Ten Speed Press.

Written by the same folks who penned *What Color Is Your Parachute*, this book includes a great discussion of the barriers individuals with disabilities may encounter when seeking employment as well as a complete explanation of the protections that the American with Disabilities Act legislation provides.

Wandro, Mark (1985).
My Daddy Is a Nurse. New York, New York: HarperCollins Juvenile Books.

This is a lovely book that describes the work of men with nontraditional men's jobs. Includes stories of a flight attendant, homemaker, dental hygienist, weaver, children's librarian, ballet dancer, preschool teacher and, yes, nurse.

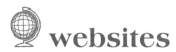

Resources

websites

American Association of Medical Professionals with Hearing Loss
www.amphl.org
This is a bright, informative site that includes an online professional journal, information on education of health-care professionals with hearing loss and information about the Association's annual conference.

Association of Nurses in AIDS Care
www.anacnet.org/leadership/hiv-nurses.htm
The ANAC offers a quarterly newsletter for HIV+ nurses and students.

Callahan's Home Online
www.callahanonline.com/index.html
John Callahan, that is. Callahan, who uses a wheelchair because of a spinal cord injury, is a widely syndicated cartoonist who (in his words) "likes to let the air out of the world when it gets too full of itself." Many of Mr. Callahan's cartoons deal rather irreverently with issues of disability. On his site, you can view the last two weeks of the cartoons he has created.

Disability Right Education and Defense Fund
www.dredf.org
The DREDF was founded in 1979 by people with disabilities and parents of children with disabilities. This site is the home page for the DREDF, which is a national law and policy center dedicated to protecting and advancing the civil rights of people with disabilities. Includes information such as articles and a newsletter about the legal rights of individuals with disabilities, mostly written in easy to understand language. Also includes information about international law as it relates to employment of folks with disabilities.

Exceptional Nurse
www.exceptionalnurse.com
ExceptionalNurse.com is a resource network committed to inclusion of more people with disabilities in the nursing profession. Has loads of articles on nurses and student nurses; includes book reviews, scholarship information, message boards, and perhaps best of all, online mentoring connections between nurses with disabilities.

Gay Health
GayHealth.com
A health and wellness site targeted toward Lesbian, Gay, Bisexual and Transgendered consumers as well as health-care professionals. Has content divided into a number of sections including news, sexual health, emotional health, general health, food and fitness, etc. The site also includes a providers' forum for health-care professionals.

Male Nurse Magazine
www.malenursemagazine.com
The Website of the online only (for now) Male Nurse Magazine. Includes a job search function, stats about men in nursing and the history of men in nursing, as well as a free ezine.

Minority Nurse
www.minoritynurse.com
Minority Nurse is a portal-like career and educational resource for the minority nursing professional. Includes articles, featured stories, a job search function, information about mentoring, and scholarships. You can also sign up for their free, super-informative e-mail newsletter.

National Association of Hispanic Nurses
www.thehispanicnurse.org
Helpful information for Hispanic nurses. Includes information about upcoming and past conferences, as well as the Association's newsletter, scholarships and a chat room.

The National Black Nurses' Association
www.nbna.org
This site includes a career center, details an amazing scholarship program, and offers partial archives of the NBNA journal.

U.S. Equal Opportunity Commission
www.eeoc.gov
This is the Federal government's Equal Opportunity site, which contains an overview of federal laws related to equal opportunity, details different types of discrimination, and explains how to file a complaint. Although the site itself is beyond huge, it loads quickly thanks to a lack of obnoxious graphics.

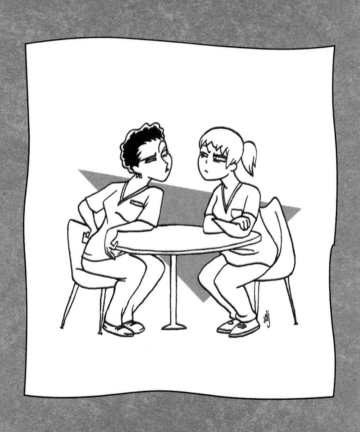

You're Not the Boss of Me (well, actually...)

A Nurse Speaks

"I've always struggled with authority, even as a kid I had that infamous 'you're not the boss of me' comment down to an art form. So when I got my first nursing job, I had some problems with my first nurse manager. I would balk at her instructions, especially when she was telling me to do something I was already on my way to do, or double-checking something that I already did. Now that I am a preceptor to new grads, I appreciate what my first nurse manager was doing and realize now that she cared enough about my professional development to help guide me."

AJ, 23-year veteran RN, New Mexico

 ## Your Preceptors

As you step onto the floor your first day at your first nursing job (or first day on any new nursing job) there will be a preceptor standing at the entrance to the unit with a smile on his or her face, eager to help teach you, guide you, and bring you into the unit fold. The preceptor will probably have made you lunch and will spend the first day complimenting your skills and making sweet "isn't this nurse brilliant" comments, accompanied by maternal clucking noises.

Or not. But you will most likely have a preceptor, or even more likely, a group of preceptors. Depending on your level of experience and the type of unit you're on, the preceptor will be assigned responsibilities such as teaching you about the particular patient population, helping you learn the policies and procedures of your facility and/or unit, guiding you into handling a full patient load, etc.

Preceptors and precepting programs vary widely from facility to facility, so perhaps the biggest trick to having a good preceptor-preceptee relationship is figuring out exactly what you are expected to learn from the time you spend with your preceptor. Usually the answer will be "function as full RN, handling a full case load while providing safe care," but hopefully your employer will provide additional, more detailed objectives, including specific clinical objectives. Although it will be difficult in the first few weeks at your position, it will be helpful if you can keep these objectives somewhere in your head (perhaps filed between "pick up new uniform" and "take dog to get spayed") because it will ultimately be your responsibility to make sure you meet them. For example, let's say one of the objectives to be completed during your precepting time is "perform a return demonstration on dressing change for patient s/p gunshot wound." If for some reason your unit (which is usually inundated with gunshot wounds, hence the objective) goes 6 weeks without having such a patient, you may need to keep your ears open for any word of a patient with a gunshot wound on the floor. Then you can volunteer to do the dressing, which will thrill both your preceptor and undoubtedly the primary nurse. Of course the patient may be less thrilled, but your preceptor will (hopefully) be right there and everyone will come through the situation just fine. Or, in the case of the patient, as fine as one can be s/p a gunshot wound.

In addition to understanding the preceptorship objectives, it's important to understand the psyche of your preceptors. Although they probably won't welcome a 45-minute cross-examination, it may be helpful to ask some (relatively) subtle questions about their background and experience so you can consider their advice and guidance in context.

As Jim Darnes, who has worked as an oncology staff nurse in Oklahoma for 2 years said, "You have to know where your preceptor is coming from to really get the best out of the experience. God help you if your preceptor was forced into service by the hospital and doesn't enjoy the preceptor role...but if that's the case, it's helpful to know that, so you don't think the short answers, maybe a little snippy attitude, is all about you. I had two preceptors when I started out: one was a little burnt out but still really really cared for the patients and the other was really very technically oriented, much more cued in to the machines, lab values, etc., than to people. They were both good nurses and I could see why the hospital chose them to be preceptors. The second nurse, especially, didn't interact with patients the way I would have, but she did teach me a lot about paying attention to concrete details. When I realized that her style just wasn't my style, I could relax a little more and still learn from her."

Jim's last comment brings us to our last comment about preceptors—

always remember that a preceptor is not a mentor. Many times floor preceptors don't even volunteer to precept, they were—as Jim said—"forced into service." They might get a big kick out of teaching new grads and nurses new to the unit, but then again they may be somewhat less enthusiastic. Make the best use of the time you have with your preceptor but don't despair if you have different nursing styles, or they are not everything you think a nurse should be.

Your Nurse Manager

Unless you lived under a rock for the years of your life until you started nursing school, you've had a boss, and undoubtedly learned, possibly through a difficult trial-and-error process, how to best work with many different types of supervisors.

It may sound like a song from the *Mr. Roger's Neighborhood*, but it's true; no two nurse managers are alike. Some supervisors are hands-on, donning scrubs and jumping into patient care when the census gets high and staffing is low. Others are extremely hands-off, and would no more don scrubs and pull a Foley than they would don a cape and attempt to fly. Some nurse managers are social and chatty and very much interested in how you spent your weekend, whereas another nurse manager might seem stumped when asked, "Hi, how are you doing?" Some nurse managers want to know everything about everything that's happening on the floor, others delegate and feel informing them about anything less than an imminent meteor landing at the nurses' station is unnecessary.

There are as many different leadership styles as there are nurse managers, and there is no one way to have a good working relationship with your supervisor. In talking with nurses for this book, however, certain types of behavior were consistently mentioned that help or hinder the nurse manager relationship. We've included a discussion of these behaviors here.

Ever walked into your front room after a long shift, thrown your keys on the hall table and turned on the light, only to have 30 people jump out and yell "surprise" at you? Perhaps this was enjoyable if it was near your birthday, anniversary, or wedding, etc. However, based on conversations we had with both nurse managers and staff nurses, very few folks like surprises outside the social party context. Nurse managers don't like to be surprised with information about a patient gone bad, or a staffing situation, or a wild jaguar being loose on the unit, etc. They, to channel Mr. Rogers again, "like to be told." And not at the last minute, i.e., when they are putting on their coat to go home, 3 minutes before a staff meeting, or when the jaguar has snuck off with the narc keys and is stealing all the Demerol, etc. Perhaps not coincidentally, staff nurses don't like to be surprised, for example (and this is an actual example) by getting a memo in their December paycheck that the customary year-end bonus is not enclosed.

Of course, patients can go bad in a moment, and it only takes a split second for that nice jaguar that came to visit Mrs. Jones to go from sweetly scary to menacing and dangerous. But when it's possible, let your nurse manager (or if more appropriate, your charge nurse) know when a situation is developing. It's natural to want to shield the person in charge from the knowledge that you might not have everything under control. At the same time, unless you've brought your stun gun, you're going to need help subduing the jaguar (be it a literal or a figurative one). Your nurse manager will ultimately appreciate the few extra minutes you give her to log on to howtosubdueawildanimalinthehospitalnenvironment.com before the situation becomes an actual emergency.

Another tip nurses mentioned for getting along with nurse managers is never head to their office with a problem without a proposed solution in mind. "It doesn't have to be a perfect solution or even a great one," explained Sherry Linden, an RN working in Toronto, Ontario, Canada, "but I've found if you put your cards on the table and say, 'Okay this is what's happening and I thought we might try x or maybe y,' you come off as a more constructive person. Your nurse manager—if she's any good—will listen to your complaints more carefully because she'll know you aren't just complaining for its own sake."

Finally, it's important to make peace with the fact that your nurse manager—because of his or her position—is sometimes going to have different loyalties and priorities than you do. KL, a nurse manager in an urban hospital on the West Coast of the United States, explained it this way, "When a nurse comes to me with a problem, I do my best to resolve it fairly and I try very hard to be an advocate not just for the patients on our floor but for the nurses too. At the same time, I really wish that nurses realized that I have to be accountable to the bean counters. I mean there are people upstairs that write me memos about the cost of chux and why are we using so many, etc. I try and shield the nurses from this when I can, but sometimes I give in to the pressure from upstairs because if I don't I won't have a job…and the next nurse manager might not advocate for nurses as much as I do." See A Nurse Manager Speaks for an interview we conducted with Sally Dillon, a nurse manager in a large Philadelphia hospital, who shared insights about relationships with staff nurses and other professionals from a manger's perspective.

In addition to learning to deal effectively with your nurse manager, being a successful nurse invariably requires learning to deal with doctors. For some tips on developing these skills, see Dealing with Docs.

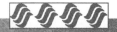

A Nurse Manager Speaks

An Interview with Sally Dillon, RN—Clinical Manager of Graduate Hospital Emergency Department, Philadelphia, Pennsylvania.

Q. How long have you been with Graduate Hospital?
A. 25 years

Q. How long have you been an RN?
A. 26 years

Q. Was it always in a managerial capacity?
A. No I have been the clinical manager of the ED for 5 years.

Q. What is your definition of an exceptional nurse-manager?
A. Someone who is a role model, a mentor open to discussion and disagreement. Someone who is able to be fair and consistent and who will promote staff development (personally and professionally).

Q. What are your thoughts on doctor/nurse relationships today?
A. I've seen a decline in the quality of relationships. The level of mutual respect seems to have diminished. Nurses are not listened to with enough genuine intent and are treated condescendingly at times. This seems especially true with young doctors who may still feel they have to have all the answers or have something to prove. Actual communication training both for nurses and doctors would be beneficial, as knowing how to approach and speak to people constructively is helpful to everyone. Without mutual tact and appreciation, vicious cycles ensue, especially during stressful scenarios. This can also be perpetuated by nurses as well.

Q. What pointers, "coping mechanisms" or strategies would you suggest to a new nurse or a nurse returning to the work-field for optimizing nurse/doctor communication and professional satisfaction?
A. The direct approach decreases miscommunication. Face to face discussion of feelings and issues is important. Of course this should be done in a private setting, not in the middle of the nurses' station, which is unprofessional and defensiveness-provoking as well. A nurse can and should demand respect, but must first do so by example. You can't demand what you're not willing to give. Also, while being assertive, make sure your statements reflect your competency level; make sure you know your level of expertise (in other words, get your facts straight).

(continued)

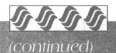
Q. *What suggestions do you have for optimizing the staff nurse/nurse manager relationship?*

A. *The direct approach again. Open communication. Avoid the rumor mill and gossip. There needs to be an ongoing open dialogue about the expectations of the unit. Managers need to remember that the people that deal with issues and the hospital's systems every day may know the best way to handle issues. Discussion about better, more efficient, etc. ways of delivering quality care, with all those who do the delivering is imperative. Staff should remember that managers don't have all the answers. A good manager promotes ownership of the unit and its collective goals and values their staff's input. Staff can help the manager to achieve as many goals as possible by genuine contribution of information. Both staff and managers should consider the concept of teamwork a priority, with issues as well as praises being conceptualized within that construct.*

Q. *Do you have a pet peeve about staff nurse/nurse manager communications?*

A. *Hearing about problems for the first time from outside sources. I don't want to hear about difficulties "through the grapevine." Staff should come first to their manager and an effort to resolve the problem within the unit can be made if appropriate. It's also possible that the manager has a more global perspective and may realize that an issue is more complex or larger than an individual or the staff realizes. More appropriate, accurate resolution may be possible if the manager is allowed to have a more informed knowledge base to start with.*

Q. *What should new nurses realistically expect from their managers?*

A. *That managers will have new or returning nurses mentored by experienced, clinically excellent RNs. Personal needs related to orientation length and perspective will be taken into consideration. Managers should remember that charting and paperwork can be overwhelming. The manager has an obligation to check in with the nurse, provide direct observation as well as feedback.*

Q. *What should they not expect?*

A. *That your manager will be able to "hold your hand" or resolve all problems. The orientee must keep in close contact with their manager and discuss issues of their own accord. Unfortunately, all requests cannot be granted. The new nurse must remember that the manager must make "universal decisions" and not only individual needs can be considered. The nursing shortage does not mean that preferential treatment can be expected. On the contrary, patients are sicker on presentation, and there is a finite amount of nurses to go around. Nursing may be rewarding but it will never be an easy job.*

(continued)

Q. Can you describe your strategy for maintaining organization and focus during a busy day on the floor?

A. Prioritize and multi-task! For example, hook up the cardiac monitor while you ask the patient's history, draw the blood at the same time as placing the IV, and so forth. As the experience in your specific specialty increases, you will know what labs and other things probably will be necessary. Draw them all at once. This save[s] your patient sticks and you time. Always do whatever you can earlier than later. If you think, "I'll have time to check my code cart later," or, "I'll do that EKG after the head C/T" you'll invariably forget or fall behind and feel overwhelmed and disorganized. Chart early and often. You have a right and responsibility to document in a timely fashion. You will never remember all the details accurately hours later and again you'll feel anxious about making omissions or mistakes. Remember to mentally note times you're doing things or observing reactions. Notes should be chronologically oriented, especially when you're in the middle of an emergency and truly can't document immediately (as during a code). Remember that you may need to be flexible and constantly reprioritize due to emergencies or changing conditions (you'll be glad for the "do everything you can early" rule here). This will include prioritizing the demands of doctors, patients, and coworkers as well. Direct communication and avoidance of passive-aggressive behaviors will become very handy at this point!

Q. What do you think about self-scheduling?

A. Staff scheduling based on unit needs and unit-staffing criteria is a good thing. Just writing in what you want to work without considering the whole picture is not. It's not an individual process. If the schedule is left with "holes," the manager must move people around to fill them. Ideally the staff should self-regulate this, but that is not always the reality.

Q. What are the most common scheduling difficulties?

A. "Holes." Rotation issues. Imbalance of staff (such as 4 on 1 dayshift and 1 on another). Balancing unit needs with ensuring staff longevity. Scheduling is extremely time consuming and one of the biggest ongoing issues.

Q. How can nurses and managers best alleviate these issues?

A. Staff can take ownership of the schedule. Make it a truly self-scheduling situation. Seniority cannot be the only factor and nurses must be "team players." Managers cannot expect that every hole will be fillable, but staff should make every effort to negotiate the schedule amongst themselves and, if necessary, with the manager, before the situation is at crisis level.

(continued)

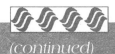

Q. *What do you see as the most challenging issue(s) for your staff nurses today?*

A. *Issues related to 'burnout,' the nursing shortage, and the aging of the nursing population. There can be a chronic stress level associated with nursing because of the pace and issues with ancillary and administrative hospital services. My perspective is the Emergency Department, and the nursing shortage has brought about further challenges for our staff because of the disruption of patient flow. In other words, patient/staff ratios are capped on the inpatient floors. The shortage has decreased nursing availability upstairs and therefore the ability of ED staff to get ED admissions upstairs. Of course there is never a "cap" in the ED and so the ED remains full. This can cause disgruntled families, uncomfortable patients, and stressed staff that feels unable to remedy the situation.*

Q. *How do you guide your staff through this issue?*

A. *Dedication, open communication and teamwork, as well as amazing people skills are what keep our nurses going. I also try to repeatedly remind my staff how much their work, expertise, and sacrifice is appreciated. I keep them as up to date as I can about company plans and policy. I keep my staff as informed as possible. Information is a powerful thing and staff needs to have as much as is available. Also, my nurses show me how much pride and how much a part of their identity being an exceptional nurse is. When I hear a nurse say, "We just saved that man's life" and I've just witnessed that truth, the importance of their "job" is obvious and the stress is worth it right then. That gives me hope!*

Q. *What is your concept or vision of nursing for the future?*

A. *What evolution of the profession would you like to see take place? I'm concerned about the replacement of professional nurses by generalized or ancillary substitutes. What effects will that have on safety and the depersonalization of patient care? I feel there has to be a deepening awareness and respect for the unique importance of the nursing profession. This will have to occur through the media, the public, doctors, and nurses themselves. To this end, the unity of nurses will have to develop further. Nurses will have to cohesively maintain professionalism and respect. Infighting will have to become a thing of the past. Just think of the AMA and consider if nursing has any lobbying or fraternal body with the same power and support. We don't and the question is why? I also think that the public as a whole has to reevaluate the sanctity of human quality of life and the concept of care. Nursing, when allowed to fulfill its philosophies, holistically cares for the entire being and allows people to feel respect and value through the most difficult of situations. This level of commitment to the human race is not only admirable, but necessary in our increasingly alienated world. I think that nursing itself will have to pool its strengths and demand that the proper value and priority be given to the nursing profession.*

Dealing with Docs

- Be aware of differing knowledge levels. In other words, "know your docs." Two first-year residents may have very different abilities and the more thoroughly you can come to know their strengths and weaknesses, the better the teamwork will be.
- Don't assume that docs remember patients. They work with patients in a different way than nurses, most often times spending much, much, much less time. They may need a refresher every time you have a conversation. It is, of course, completely annoying to have to do this, but it's better to presume the need for this refresher than to handle miscommunication problems later.
- Be super clear about what you're saying and what you want. Be 10-times clearer than you would think you would need to be, especially when dealing with the chronically sleep deprived of the profession.
- Anticipate information, orders, etc., that you will need from the doc and get it when they are on the floor, if at all possible. This is an ability that develops over time.
- Observe other nurses. If you are having a particularly hard time communicating with a certain doc, maybe someone else has found a way to make himself heard. It may be that the doc doesn't do well over the phone, etc.
- If you have to deal with a particularly difficult doc, ask another nurse to role-play (call it by a different name if 'role-play' sounds too hokey). Be aware, especially, of the effect that the presence or absence of an audience plays in your interactions. Of course, confronting someone is most appropriately done while you are alone, or at least in the least public way you can manage. But if the doc tends to get loud/abusive, etc., she has chosen to make the discussion public and you might want to arrange the discussion so that you have witnesses.

The Evaluation Process

Even if you are a traditional-age new grad and only worked summers as a camp counselor, you've probably been through at least a semi-formal evaluation as part of a job. Nursing evaluations (aka performance reviews) are not all that different from those done for other types of employment. Many times a preliminary review is required before you are considered finished with your initial "probationary" period, and most often are done every 6 months or 1 year after that. It's helpful to ask about the evaluation criteria long before you're scheduled for your first evaluation so you know what kind of goals you're working toward.

Most facilities require the employee and the supervisor to fill out identical evaluation forms that are then compared during the evaluation meeting. Filling out the form can be somewhat perplexing especially when you're asked to provide, for example, a 1 to 5 numerical rating of your ability to "put patients at ease" or some other subjective skill. One way to add to the accuracy and meaningfulness of these types of self-ratings is to include examples or comments when possible. For example, if there is a question about "ability to handle difficult situations" (this is an example; an actual eval form would ask a more position-specific question), you could include an example of an actual incident that you helped de-escalate (leaving patient names out, of course), what types of skills you demonstrated, etc. It's especially important to include additional information and examples when the individual doing the evaluation has not had the chance to observe your work firsthand (e.g., if you work night shift and the nurse manager is only at the hospital 7 a.m.—3 p.m.).

In an ideal situation, there are no surprises during your evaluation meeting because you've been receiving feedback about your performance all along. If you are first told of a significant deficiency in a performance evaluation, it's perfectly reasonable to say, "Why wasn't I informed of this problem before now," although if you can think of a less confrontational way to say it, that might get a better response. It could be that the nurse manager thought you had been informed of a problem when you hadn't, or that there is some confusion about expectations. In such a case, it is reasonable to ask that the confusion about expectations be written into the comments section of the eval (if the nurse manager won't write it on the employer copy, you can write in it yours). Also make sure that any area that is identified as needing improvement is in included in your goals to accomplish before the next performance evaluation. In this way, anyone looking at your file can see you're making an effort to address any problems.

At the end of the evaluation, you will be asked to sign a copy of your evaluation before it is placed into your personnel record. You don't have to agree with everything in the evaluation, you are only signing that you have read it. In the event that you don't agree with something in the evaluation and you can't come to an agreement with your nurse manager, you have the option of appealing what is written by taking it to the next person in the chain of command.

 The Magic of Mentoring

Whether you just finished your last exam for nursing school yesterday or you were in Ms. Nightingale's first graduating class, you can benefit from a mentoring relationship, both as a mentor or a mentee.

How can a mentoring relationship help you? In many ways, depending on what kind of career assistance you're looking for. Mentors can be a sounding board when you need a professional to vent your professional frustrations to. A mentor can help you get your ideas and concerns noticed and taken seriously, and a mentor might know about resources for professional growth that you might be unaware of. For new grads, especially, a mentor can be an energizing force, someone to help you through the oh-my-God-I-am-so-exhausted-I-have-to-go-right-home-and-sleep-after-work syndrome (also known as new grad pseudo narcolepsy). A mentor might be a cheerleader, a challenger, or a coach.

Even if you're not a new grad, you can still benefit from a mentor, especially if you are changing positions, returning to school, or feeling stuck in a proverbial rut.

Why would someone want to be a mentor? Mentoring can be valuable for both parties. Just seeing the nursing world through new grad eyes can be an interesting and (dare we say it) inspirational experience.

Where can you find a mentor? You can find potential mentors at your workplace, former clinical sites, during nursing conventions, through online connections (for example, through minoritynurse.com or exceptionalnurse.com), or where you do volunteer work.

Before you approach a potential mentor, think about what you're asking. What is it that you want out of the relationship? You probably wouldn't feel comfortable asking a mentor to come live at your house and make sure you are roused for your 7 a.m. shift (and this does seem a bit more like babysitting than mentoring), but you could ask for a once-a-month chat over coffee, an ongoing e-mail correspondence, or to talk on the phone once a week. The clearer you can be about your expectations, about both the time you would want and what type of support you're looking for, the better your potential mentor can evaluate your request. It's hard not to feel shy about asking what we might see as a big favor, but think about the first time a patient asked you a question and you actually knew the answer. Didn't that feel great? It's human nature to want to share knowledge; you may well be meeting your mentor's needs as much as your own, especially if you demonstrate an eagerness to work toward your goals and apply what you've learned from your mentor to your own practice.

If all this sounds too much like fifth grade (i.e., when we would pass notes to potential friends that said, "Would you be my best friend, check yes or no") for your taste, you don't necessarily need some kind of formal mentoring situation, complete with a notarized form that promises mentor/mentee allegiance until death does you part. It's equally valuable to have informal mentoring relationships with nurses that you admire. You can also make a deal with another nurse to be a (and we know this sounds corny but go with us here) growth partners. For example, if you both are interested in going back to school but haven't yet made a move to do so, you can meet weekly to monitor each other's progress. As human beings we don't much care for embarrassment; never underestimate the power of a little friendly accountability.

Finally, remember that a mentor doesn't need to have the same career goals as you or even share the same specialty area. For example, one of the authors (Kelli) worked closely with a nurse who was an extremely hard worker and also an exceptional vacation planner, who through careful planning was able to traverse the world during her time off. From this nurse Kelli learned the fine art of actually using one's vacation, not to mention using it well! Kelli feels this has made her a better nurse when she comes back to work, and has helped her to love, not only her nursing career, but (no surprise here) her life as a nurse.

When You're in Charge

If you are an RN in today's wonderful world of health, unless you are extremely clever with avoidance tactics, at some point you are going to end up supervising someone, perhaps even your first day on the job. Add to this the fact that not all nursing programs fit a leadership/management course into their curriculum and this whole "Hey! I'm in charge?!" thing can be pretty overwhelming.

Don't despair though. Even if you've never been the boss, you've probably had many different bosses. If you think about what kind of communication, working environment, etc., helped you be the best employee you could be, you'll find that many other people will probably flourish under similar conditions.

Of course, you're never going to be supervising or be a charge nurse in a vacuum (where would everyone fit anyway?) so you'll have to deal with different temperaments and pre-existing conditions, not to mention the interplay of the many different types of personalities of all the people on that shift that particular day.

It helps to learn about temperament and the way temperament affects the way people interact. If you can make time (in between running for call lights, juggling emergencies, changing dressings, etc.) it's sometimes an interesting exercise to have everyone who works on the unit complete the Myers-Briggs personality assessment and then have a informal meeting to talk about the differences in results. This can not only help employees be better informed about the interaction preferences of their coworkers, it can also remind us that temperament differences are just that—differences—rather than grievous character flaws.

Understanding this can help decrease the likelihood that we'll punish our coworkers for not interacting in exactly the same manner we do.

And since we're sure you have loads of free time (ha!), it might also help if you can fit a leadership or management course into your schedule. Push your employer to pay for it! Courses are available through continuing nursing education providers, local community colleges, or even through the business world (e.g., chamber of commerce or local small business association). Unless you plan to make the study of the philosophy of leadership a lifelong goal, steer away from theoretically based courses and concentrate on finding a class that includes lots of role-play, discussion of actual scenarios, etc. Even if you don't end up permanently as charge nurse or working five decades as a nurse manager, the skills you'll learn can help you in any leadership position or when working with patients.

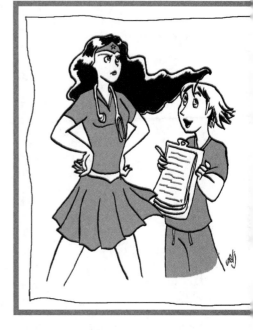

Ideally, if you're going to be assuming leadership functions on your floor/unit/department, etc., these responsibilities will be given to you gradually with a sizable amount of adjustment time allowed before assuming another new responsibility. Okay, okay, that's enough hysterical laughter. C'mon, you do agree that's the ideal, right? Anyway, if you're in a position to negotiate for a gradual taking-on of a leadership role, that's fantastic. If not, you may be suddenly placed in a situation where you're in charge, but know quite a bit less than the people you're supervising. See Jen Borek's A New Grad Speaks for her experiences in being charge nurse on her floor.

Classically, this happens to new RN grads who take jobs in long-term care. "I was supervising LPNs on my first week on the job," said Jill Glass, who graduated from a Pennsylvania BSN program last year. "I was bumbling around, trying to make up assignments, coordinate meds etc, and having to ask 'um, yeah, where is that clean linen closet anyway.' " Nurses who have experienced these situations say blatant honesty is definitely the best policy. Glass explains, "At first I wanted to cover up what a neophyte I was. But those LPNs—who were all at least twenty

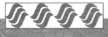

Monday, July 14, 2003

This is the start of my third week on night shift. I really like it. I have always been a night owl so the transition has not been hard at all. My family has been really great about letting me sleep during the day. I am assigned to 4S as charge nurse. Tonight was a full moon, and it showed. We had one patient in the hall in a geri chair. She was dialing her hand and asking someone to come pick her up. Then we had a woman saying the rosary with a sheet over her head. Her roommate was yelling at her sister to lock the doors and go to bed. There was no one in the room. Finally, towards the end of the shift, a patient who had asked for pain meds six times put on his call bell. When I entered his room, he looked at me and quietly asked, could you scratch my back? A nurse's job is never done.

Tuesday, July 15, 2003

Tonight was crazier than last night. I was on 4S orienting to charge again. The sweet lady saying the rosary from last night did nothing but scream all night tonight. I had about a million meds to give and 18 chart checks. My night flew by.

Wednesday, July 16, 2003

I got a call at 7:15 from the 3–11 nursing supervisor. Someone had been injured on the floor where I was due at 11 p.m. and she wondered if I could come in now. I got there before 8 p.m. and took over a primary care assignment. I picked up 5 patients including a fresh post-op. Before I knew it, it was 11 p.m. Now my regular shift started and I was in charge. I was busy all night with meds and chart checks. It was time for 6 a.m. meds before I knew it.

Thursday, July 17, 2003

Every night that I have been orienting to charge I try to modify my routine to save time. I have founds that I can do IV rounds when I pass midnight meds. I take any advice I can get from the other nurses on what time savers they had discovered that work. I was so excited that tonight I was done meds and ready for chart checks by 12:30 a.m.. Then the call came, you're getting an admission in 18A and 18B. Well, so much for a break tonight. I have been very lucky that all of my admissions thus far have been from the ER where there is a great unit clerk who takes off all of the orders. She was off tonight. At 6:20 when I had put in the last of the 28 orders 18B, I started my morning rounds.

(continued)

Friday, July 18, 2003

Ah, the end of the week. I am really looking forward to the weekend. I have so much to do at home. Tonight I was charge nurse on 4S. I answered a call for a patient who had a total knee replacement and needed pain meds. She asked if she could have a Tylenol. I looked on her Kardex and saw that she had an order for Percocet. I offered her a Percocet and she said she would take one. Two hours later she put her call bell on. I found her sitting up in bed wide awake. She told me that this was not her room. She then proceeded to tell me that this was a dirty trick I was playing on her. I thought about what they had taught us in school. Reorient the patient. Well that didn't work. After several attempts to reorient her, I apologized for switching her room. This satisfied her and she went to sleep. When I discussed this in report the day nurses had a similar experience the day before. Hello...maybe she should have a plain Tylenol order! Talk about a break in communication.

Monday, July 21, 2003

Tonight I was pulled to 2E, a telemetry floor that does primary care. I had five patients and provided all of their care. It was a nice change of pace. The patients were all on monitors which made me a little nervous. The regular staff was really nice and helped me with the cardiac documentation. I am really getting a lot of experience floating to the different floors. I hope this will prepare me for when I'm on my own.

Tuesday, July 22, 2003

Tonight, something happened that I still can't believe. I made a med error. I was in charge and giving the midnight meds for the floor. A post-op patient needed to be medicated for pain. I looked at the Kardex, he had an order for Percocet PO and Demerol IM. I went in and asked him if he wanted a shot or a tablet. He told me that his pain was really bad so he'd take the shot. No problem. I went back to the cart. Signed out the Demerol, opened the drawer got out a Dilaudid, signed the Dilaudid out on the Narc sheet and went in and gave the patient his IM injection. I went on giving meds. When I had finished, I went back like I always do and make sure I didn't miss anyone and that I signed everything out. I looked to make sure that I signed out all of the narcs and that is when I saw one Dilaudid signed out. Oh my God, I gave him Dilaudid. I almost threw up. I wanted to die. I told my preceptor and she and I called the nursing supervisor and the house doctor and filled out an incident report. In the end the patient was fine. I was so upset. When I told the nurse manager in the morning she was great. She said, I bet you'll never make that mistake again!

Wednesday, July 23, 2003

Tonight I was in charge again. I still have not recovered from my mishap last night. It took me forever to give meds because I checked everything fifty times. My preceptor told me that anyone who tells you that they have never made a mistake is lying. She said that the mistakes you made as a new nurse are from inexperience and those that you made as a seasoned nurse are because you are too comfortable. This was very reassuring. Everyone I told had a story to share. One nurse accidentally pulled out a CVP line putting up the side rails. Safety first!

(continued)

Thursday, July 24, 2003

More of the same. I was in charge tonight. There is so much to keep straight. I look at the other nurses I work with and wonder how I'll ever do what they do. I have found that I am learning more from the people I am working with, RNs, LPNs, and aides alike, than I ever did in school. Nursing is a career in which you never stop learning. There are always new ways of doing things, different ways of dealing with situations, or handling people that no text book or nursing lab could ever prepare you for.

Friday, July 25, 2003

I can't believe it has been 6 weeks. Tonight was my last night of orientation. My preceptor was off tonight so I took a primary care assignment. I am really looking forward to next week when I am on my own. There are so many changes in the works at the hospital. They are building a new wing, charging the computer system, and even trying to change the nursing model. I guess I am being idealistic, but I can't imagine ever being bored with this. There is so much to do and even more to learn. It is still hard to believe that I am a nurse. It seems like yesterday that I was applying to nursing school and now here I am. It has been an exciting journey, but I think the real excitement lies ahead.

years older than me—kept giving me these looks. Finally I said 'okay, this is really awkward because I have some responsibilities here and clearly I don't have a lot of experience on this unit or even in nursing in general. So, how can we work together and what do you need from me to [be] able to do your job?' It helps that I have real respect for the work that LPNs do, I didn't treat them as some kind of glorified bedpan chambermaids, like I have seen some RNs do."

Of course, it's a fine line between being approachable and maintaining an air of confidence so that the other folks on the floor don't have to worry about their patients and about you. Remember how you felt when you gave your first IM or suctioned your first trach? Did you feel confident? Nope, but the patient still voluntarily let you do it (well, if they were conscious anyway), most likely because you had decided (or your clinical instructor had strong-armed you into) acting in a confident manner. As the old 12-step saying goes, sometimes you've got to "fake it until you make it."

In addition, learning the science—and the art—of delegation is essential. In fact, even if you are not the charge nurse, as an RN you are going to be essentially "in charge" of other folks, usually unlicensed assistive personnel. Here's where experience (gained either on the floor or through role-playing) can come in handy, along with knowing not only your Nurse Practice Act but also your facility's policy and procedure book backwards and forwards, upside down, sideways, and, well, you get the picture.

Communication and reading cues—as well as being aware of cues you're sending out—can make a difference between a good and bad day in charge. "Sometimes you hear nurses say they don't 'play politics' but if you're dealing with people you are 'being political.' You have to have some level of social acumen," said TJ, a Texas RN who often serves as third-shift charge nurse at the long-term care facility where he works. "It's simple things like some people like to be greeted when they first come into work and some people would rather you grunt at them until they've have a chance to hit the coffee machine a few times. Not bombarding people when they first walk in is so critical to the tone of the whole shift, yet we've all known charge nurses that try to give assignments when a nurse is still taking off their coat."

Finally, nurses we talked with also agreed about one fundamental truth of being in charge. "Invariably," said Laura Lau, a 23-year veteran BSN, "people will sometimes be mad at you. You simply have to deal with that fact. As nurses we are people pleasers, but as long as you're making decisions that affect people, not everyone is going to be pleased. You have to do your best and realize you've done your best and even if everyone's not thrilled, you've helped make the shift the best you could within the limits of your control."

Resources

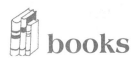 **books**

Pachter, Barbara (2000).
The Power of Positive Confrontation. New York: NY: Marlowe and Company.

Useful guide to setting boundaries and confronting difficult situations and people. Clearly written with the business world in mind, nurses may find it helpful as it explains some of the social and cultural factors that can contribute to directness or indirectness in communication.

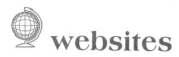

Resources

websites

Crab Bucket Rescue
www.crabbucketrescue.com
Did you hear the one about the crab who tried to get out of the bucket? No? Hit this site and learn about abandoning ineffective ways of thinking to increase your leadership effectiveness. Includes book reviews and great articles. Don't miss the extremely cute (animated even) crab graphics.

The Keirsey Temperament Sorter
www.keirsey.com
Although this site can be a little confusing to use, it's the best free site we've found for "sorting" (their word) temperaments. A little self-knowledge can be a powerful thing!

National Association of Directions of Nursing Administration in Long-Term Care
www.nadona.org
Behind this seemingly unassuming little Website lurks a veritable cornu-copia of information. Some is specific to long-term care administration but most is valuable to any nurse who has any charge responsibilities. You can read some articles from their publication The Director online as well as get information about their annual conference.

Nursing Management
www.nursingmanagement.com
This is the online home of *Nursing Management* a monthly journal of prac-tical information for nurse leaders. Includes a wide range of topics, such as legal and ethical aspects of nursing leadership, personnel management, recruitment and retention, budget issues, product selection, and quality control.

Nurturing Your Success Home Page
www.nurturingyourscucess.com
This site is the online home of Nurturing Your Success Coaching and Financial Advisement Services. The treasure here is tons of articles, many on management issues including the art of prioritizing, delegation, and embracing change.

Work Ethics Wizard
Workethicswizard.com
At this site you can sign up for a free e-zine about managing people for best productivity. Site is bright and easy to read

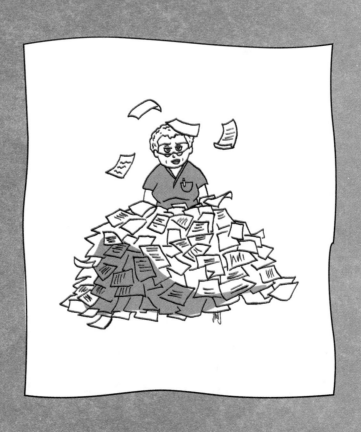

9

CHAPTER

Legal and Ethical Issues

A Nurse Speaks

Like everyone else, I'm afraid of being sued, but in the current healthcare climate, I don't see how it can be avoided. As long as facilities keep substituting unlicensed assistive personnel for RNs, as long as they keep pushing staff to the limits, I think there are going to be lots of lawsuits. My hope is to cover myself well enough that I'm not personally implicated. I just wish I knew more about how to do that."

MP, 12-year veteran RN, MN

Few things are more anxiety provoking for nurses than conversations that involve the word "legal" and the word "concerns." In fact, just writing this chapter made us a little anxious.

This is, of course, a natural reaction. None of us wants to be involved in any sort of adversarial interaction, either within the facility where we work or from the outside (i.e., a litigious patient or family member).

As in any situation that provokes anxiety, we can try to swallow the anxiety (not exactly the most effective tactic) or we can use the anxiety to motivate us to action. In the case of legal concerns, this could mean seeking out articles about risk management or attending continuing education programs that address charting and liability or even something you're already doing...like reading this chapter!

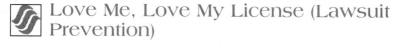 Love Me, Love My License (Lawsuit Prevention)

If Smokey the Bear ran the risk-management department at your hospital, he might say, "Only you can prevent a lawsuit," in his half-pleading, half-authoritative way. Fortunately, I suppose for us, Smokey the Bear is too busy with his anti–forest fire activism to moonlight. So hopefully, the folks in charge at your facility realize that lawsuit prevention is not just you (or any one nurse)—it's a team effort.

The facility's part in lawsuit prevention involves responsibilities such as adequate maintenance of the physical plant, providing appropriate infrastructure so that patient needs can be met, and perhaps most importantly, adequate staffing. Of course, if the institution doesn't provide these things, it's still your responsibility not only to give safe patient care but also to hold the institution responsible for its irresponsibility. We'll discuss ways to hold institution responsible later in the chapter, but first we'll discuss what you as an individual can do to prevent lawsuits.

Laws vary from state to state and because we're not lawyers, we are not going to write about specific situations or scenarios that may or may not expose a nurse (and his or her facility) to disciplinary action, lawsuits, civil or criminal charges, etc.

There are however, some general types of actions and situations that are more likely than others to trigger lawsuits and we do want to examine these, so you can avoid them and make your practice as lawsuit-proof as possible.

You might be thinking, "Okay authors, I've been going along with you thus far, but I don't need to read this section. I know what triggers lawsuits—mistakes and bad outcomes. It's not exactly rocket science."

True that, dear reader, but even in our extremely litigious society, not all dissatisfied health-care consumers initiate a lawsuit and not everyone who initiates a lawsuit has had an actual poor outcome.

So, clearly there are other influencing factors. In addition to providing excellent care, understanding and attempting to control these factors (when possible) can decrease the possibility that you'll one day find yourself staring down the wrong end of a subpoena.

Vincent, Young, and Phillips (1994) researched why patients (and family) initiate legal action. They found four major reasons:

1. Accountability, feeling like staff members should be disciplined and made to "pay" for their actions
2. Explanation, wanting an explanation, especially if the patient felt ignored or neglected after an incident
3. Standards of care—wanting to prevent a future incident of the same type
4. Compensation—wanting to be compensated for what they have experienced

Thinking about these main themes can inform your actions and attitudes when dealing with a difficult situation or patient. For example, an extremely common cause of litigation (the most common, if you draw your conclusion from legal commercials on daytime TV) involves a patient fall.

We all know patients fall. Some of these falls are justifiably preventable. But in certain situations, falls are extremely difficult to prevent, and in some situations, the actions of patients/family members contribute to the fall (i.e., an unstable patient who insists on getting out of bed without assistance, a family that refuses sedation or restraint when it is temporarily needed to help a confused patient stay safe). Yet, regardless of the cause, once the patient is on the floor and the damage is done (in either the form of actual harm or the impression of harm), there might be several ways to mitigate the likelihood of a lawsuit.

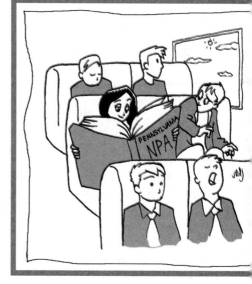

According to G.W. Guido's *Legal and Ethical Issues in Nursing* (2001), most research revealed that actions such as treating the patient and family members honestly, respectfully, and openly, as well as expressing compassion, can help a nurse avoid legal problems. In this case, it might mean sincerely expressing regret for the patient's fall (you can make a compassionate statement without admission of wrongdoing if you are worried about your words being used against you later) or taking the time to let a family member vent feelings about the fall. Of course, these actions are really just good nursing care, but going the extra mile on these occasions may really pay off in the end.

A number of nurses we talked with about these type of situations suggested that especially when situations involve multiple staff members, if there's one staff member who is particularly adept at handling difficult situations or angry people, make sure that staff member takes the lead on the patient/family interaction. On the other hand, we all have coworkers whose lack of social skills (or more commonly, personal insecurity) often leads to an escalation of whatever situation is at hand. Many, many, many nurses mentioned these types of folks and strongly suggested that they should be kept away from the sticky situations we've talked about, perhaps even—as one nurse jokingly suggested—"locked in the clean linen closet until the end of the shift."

Rules, Rules, Rules: The Nurse Practice Act and You

Even if you're a new grad, by now you're familiar with a little thing called the Nurse Practice Act. The Nurse Practice Act is what governs the um, practice of nursing in your state (clever, huh?), although in a few states it's called by an ever so slightly different name. A Nurse Practice Act—even known by any other name—is just as important for nurses to read and understand. Unfortunately, practice acts tend to be both rather lengthy and written in legalese. This explains why it's much more common to see someone reading a Stephen King novel instead of a Nurse Practice Act on the bus.

Most states allow you to download from their Website an electronic copy of the Nurse Practice Act or will provide you with a written copy (usually for a fee, of course). Procuring a copy is a good start but to understand the act and what it means to your daily practice, it's helpful to take an explanatory class. Don't panic (or scoff!). We're talking about a day-long training or a seminar, not a three-credit graduate course. Some boards of nursing offer these types of classes, you might also be able to find them through organizations that offer continuing nursing education, through your employer (check with the department of nursing or risk management), or through your state nursing organization. Seminars on how the Nurse Practice Act applies to your individual specialty area may also be available during your specialty area's convention, although the guidelines given will tend to be more general since the presenter will most likely be dealing with individuals from multiple states.

Another good source of information about the Nurse Practice Act and other matters related to legal concerns is organizations that issue nursing malpractice insurance policies. Which reminds us to ask, you do have malpractice insurance, right? Right?

Two words: get it. We know your institution has its own insurance, but you can't trust their insurance company to be looking out for you first. Not only that, if you do any type of volunteer work (and guess what, taking an elderly neighbor's blood pressure counts) you'll want the non–work-based coverage. Plus, it's really cheap. The cost of a year of comprehensive nursing malpractice insurance for the average staff nurse is less than 20% of what liability insurance costs for someone who teaches scuba diving.

 ## Assignment Despite Objection

Okay, you've done your part. You're involved in continuing education so that your nursing practice is current (and therefore, more likely to be safe). You've read, studied, and re-read your state's Nurse Practice Act (maybe even on the bus). You're a kind compassionate soul who has learned how to handle families in crisis and you keep your socially inept coworkers out of the way when potentially litigious trouble is brewing. You are now 100% safe from a lawsuit, right?

Unfortunately, (and unfairly) that's not quite accurate. There's a little factor called "all the stuff your employer does" that can contribute to lawsuit potential.

Thanks to many factors, including decreased Medicare and Medicaid reimbursements not to mention corporate greed, health-care providing institutions are under more pressure than ever to cut costs. It apparently would be ludicrous to expect health-care chain CEOs to take commercial air flights instead of jetting around in their own company plane. So, instead, one extremely common way institutions try to save money is by reducing the cost of staffing.

Institutions attempt to do this in a number of ways and most of them are nightmares for nurses (not to mention patients). Floating, mandatory overtime, reducing staff, relegating responsibilities formerly assigned to RNs to unlicensed assistive personnel are a few examples. All these have the potential to cause situations that are unsafe for both staff and patients.

Ideally, as you chose an employer you've considered the impact of any current cost-cutting measures the facility already has in place. But as long as there are company jets and company yachts to purchase, there's always the chance you'll come to work one day to find all your fellow nurses in the break room gathered around a memo entitled "New Mandatory RN Floating Policy."

Such memos are the stuff of which nightmares are made (such memos along with watching local TV news too close to bedtime) but don't despair just yet.

Talk with your union rep or nursing manager (or better yet, both) about what the changes mean. A new floating policy that's instituted with an extensive cross-training program is going to affect you a lot differently than one that is accompanied by a training program that consists of a memo instructing you to "get out your old nursing school textbooks and read up on…everything."

If you feel the new policy is going to create unsafe situations, band together with your fellow nurses to confront the powers that be. If you have a union, that's the obvious place to start, but if necessary contact your state nurses' organization, which may be able to provide you with valuable information about the best way to advocate against the new policy.

Despite your best-informed employment decision and efforts to change potentially unsafe staffing policies, you may find yourself in a situation where you are asked to provide care in a situation that is clearly not safe.

Walking away from the assignment leaves you open to charges of patient abandonment, which could potentially lead to loss of licensure as well as even criminal prosecution.

It's for these types of situations that the Assignment Despite Objection form was created. The Assignment Despite Objection (hereafter ADO) form is not a magical "get out of jail free" card; just filing an ADO doesn't guarantee, well, anything. As a professional, you are still legally liable for the care you give, regardless of the situation. Nevertheless, the ADO form is useful because it creates a paper trail and holds systems responsible for the unsafe situations the system creates. This paper trail can then be used as supportive documentation in arguments to improve staffing, either in contract negotiations with individual institutions or in support of legislation.

The ADO form is available either from your union rep or from your state nurses' association. The form itself varies, but typically asks for such information as the census, the acuity of patients, staffing numbers, and the specific objection of the nurse (e.g., inadequate staff, too few RNs, not oriented to unit, not trained or experienced in areas assigned). There is also usually a space for comments. Note that part of the process for completing an ADO form is informing your immediate supervisor you feel the situation is unsafe and asking for a change. When you give them a copy of the ADO form they shouldn't be surprised! Although the distribution of the ADO varies, the form itself will have instructions on how many copies to make, where to send them, etc. Usually the procedure is a copy for your personal file, one to your nursing supervisor, one to the local union head (if applicable), and another to your state nurses' organization or the local representative.

Ethics in the Workplace

Ah, ethics, another relaxing topic.

It's almost a truism to say that nurses are surrounded with ethical issues every day because, in fact, everyone is surrounded with ethical issues every day. But as nurses we are extremely trusted members of society and also have a great deal of personal contact with individuals who are very vulnerable in a number of ways. Having a thought-out, informed ethical framework from which we make decisions is imperative for us.

The structure for the profession's ethical expectations is found in the American Nurses Associations Code for Nurses with Interpretative Statement. You can view the Code on-line at the ANA site (http://nursingworld.org/ethics/code/ethicscode150.htm). If you want a hard copy, you have to buy one from the ANA site because they've set it up so you can't print it from the Web (and no, you can't copy and paste it into a new text document, we tried that, too).

Anyway, however you get your hands on it, read it! The Code isn't set up like a Nurses' Ten Commandments with a series of specific "thou shall" or "thou shall nots." Instead, it contains a series of nine provisions with their accompanying interpretive statements. The first three provisions address the most basic commitments and values of the nurse; the second three address the issues of boundaries and loyalty, and the last three address the duties of nursing as a whole (i.e., beyond individual patient encounters). The nine provisions are changed less often than the interpretive statements, which address more specific possibilities in practice and are updated more frequently to reflect the context of nursing as it exists at the time of the revision.

If you want more specific ethical guidelines, the ANA also publishes policy statements that provide the ANA position on clinical, research and public policy issues. These are also available on the ANA site.

If you are having a particular ethical dilemma, there are a few places you can get answers to questions. Many facilities (especially if they are part of a larger system) have hotlines where you can speak to an ethics specialist (usually anonymously, but check first) about a specific situation. If your facility doesn't offer a hotline, you may still be able to talk to someone on the ethics committee; a peruse through the hospital director will yield their contact info.

References

American Nurses Association. (2001). Code of Ethics for Nurses with Interpretive Statements,. American Nurses Publishing: Washington, D.C.

Guido, G.W. (2001). Legal and Ethical Issues In Nursing. Appleton and Lange: Stamford, CT.

Vincent, C., Young, M. & Phillips, A. (1994). Why do people sue doctors? A study of patients and relatives taking legal action. *Lancet, 343,* 1609–1613.

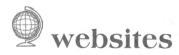 **websites**

American Nurses Association Center for Ethics and Human Rights
www.nursingworld.org/ethics/center
This is the spot on the Web where the ANA Code of Ethics resides.

Nursing Law On-Line
www.nursinglaw.com
At this site you can read a sample issue of the *Legal Eagle Eye Newsletter for the Nursing Profession*, which focuses on nurses' professional negligence, employment, discrimination, and licensing issues.

Virtual Nurse
www.virtualnurse.com
Links, links, links. This site is a collection of many different nursing links, many to the home pages of Legal Nurse Consultants.

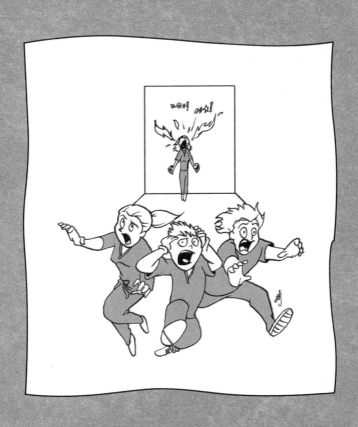

10

The Mess That Is Stress

A Nurse Speaks:

"I've recognized burnout [from stress] more than once in myself. I don't want to go to work anymore and when I'm there I want to leave as fast as I can. I get depressed in my life away from work and then I know it's time to either change my job or change my attitude or do what I can within the context of the job to fix it. There are always options, but a lot of nurses can't see them when they're in the midst of burnout."

Kathryn Cantley, RN

"Stress" has become such an overused word that it has all but lost its meaning in our modern society. In fact, when you hear someone say "I'm stressed" they might mean anything from "I would very much prefer to be napping in a field of daisies right now" to "I am 30 seconds away from purchasing an automatic weapon with which to start Armageddon."

So how do we define stress? We're quite glad you asked. For the purposes of our discussion (and borrowing from the nursing adage about pain) we offer this definition: stress is whatever a particular individual finds anxiety provoking, and it's as anxiety provoking to them as they say it is. For example, some nurses would rather eat a snow cone made of glass shavings than participate in a code, others find the challenge and action exhilarating. One nurse might like the autonomy of the night shift; another nurse might find that no amount of autonomy of practice can compensate for having to work while the rest of the world sleeps. What you find stressful at work can also be affected by where you are in your career. Many new grads we talked with stated they felt "very stressed" when taking care of a patient with an unfamiliar diagnosis, nurses with more experience more often found this a welcome change in routine. And since nurses do have a life outside of work (no matter what the occasional nurse manager seems to think), stress doesn't stop at the hospital door.

Stress is not always—as we all learned in nursing school—a terrible thing, nor is it only a result of terrible things happening to us. Even positive events can be stressful. What could cause more stress than the last push that launches a laboring woman's baby into the world? Yet, if the baby is a desired addition to her life, the stress of the moment will undoubtedly seem worth the effort.

In addition, it's stress—or at least tension—that gets us out of bed in the morning and in general helps us fulfill our commitments when perhaps we'd rather do something else. For example, in those moments when we don't feel like being particularly responsible and would rather buy an adorable embroidered gold lame vest for our new puppy instead of paying our rent, the stressful thought of being evicted and living with our new puppy on the street, helps us make a more positive choice.

In general, a healthy human being can handle the load of some stress. But when we encounter multiple stressors within a short time, lack positive ways to deal with stress, or encounter stressful situations without support, we can all suffer ill effects. In this chapter, we share positive techniques for understanding and coping with stress that have worked for us or the nurses we interviewed.

Good Fences Make Good Neighbors: Boundaries and You

For nurses, one of the most effective stress management tools is setting and maintaining effective boundaries. Boundaries, simply put, are limits, particularly limits on what you are or aren't willing to do for other people and ways in which you feel comfortable interacting with others.

Boundaries are our lifeline, in fact they make our work as nurses possible. Every day nurses work with suffering people in a way that goes even beyond "up close and personal." And since any individual with so much as a modicum of compassion wants to alleviate suffering when possible, we naturally want to keep helping more and more, giving more and more (and more…and more…and more) of ourselves in the process. The problem with this tendency however, is that if we let our work completely take over our personal lives, or if we let our patients' problems and suffering become our own, it will eventually make us miserable and will also make a long-term nursing career nigh unto unsustainable.

As nurses, we sometimes find it difficult to set and defend boundaries, for many reasons, not the least of which is we sometimes feel that having rigid rules will make us rigid nurses. It's important to remember that boundaries are not walls that we create to cut ourselves off emotionally from patients as much as possible or to enable us to hide behind our professional façade. On the contrary, having good, reasonable limits about what we can reasonably do and what we will reasonably tolerate, enables us to give freely from within.

Or as one experienced nurse who identified herself as "in recovery from having NO boundaries" said, "Without boundaries, you have no way to keep every bit of your life force from being taken from you. It's like some kind of scene from a B horror flick 'the Nurse Whose Soul Was Sucked Out.' But with boundaries, you can help people without hurting yourself."

Of course, there are the basic boundaries that a nurse, in all fairness, should not have to ask to be respected. All workplaces (well, all places in general!) should be physical, sexual, and emotional abuse-free zones, but this is not always the case. In fact, many of the nurses with whom we talked had encountered at least one of these types of abuse on the job. A Texas RN summed it up best when she said, "As nurses we encounter—and tolerate—abusive situations that folks in other professions would never tolerate. In a situation [involving abuse] when someone else would already be on the phone with a union rep, a lawyer, a therapist, and the local paper, a nurse might still be at the 'hmmm. I don't know if I feel comfortable with that' stage."

It's way beyond the scope of this chapter to address the cultural and social reasons why abusive situations may be more common in nursing than other professions. There are some excellent resources listed at the end of this chapter that cover this topic in depth. But for the individual nurse who may be working in a situation where abuse is tolerated, or even worse, considered part of the job, it would be easy for us to sit here in book-writing land and say, "Get out! Leave! Don't look back!" But we also know there are a myriad of reasons why a nurse might not feel free to leave an abusive workplace, not the least of which is concern about finances. We would suggest nurses who are in these situations make use of some of the resources listed at the end of this chapter to help them decide how to proceed.

In some situations, deciding if a situation is really 'abusive" can be quite difficult because any profession involves an element of risk and working with patients who might not be completely cognitively aware presents other ambiguities. For example, a nurse working in an ER might consider sometimes having to deal with combative patients a reasonable occupational risk. But if the hospital routinely fails to provide appropriate safeguards (e.g., adequate security, sufficient staff, training in the use of restraints), the same situation might be considered abusive. In another case, most nurses would agree that if a physician touched a nurse in a sexual (and non-consensual) way that would be sexually abusive. But what if the touch is attempted by a patient who recently suffered frontal lobe damage as the result of a traumatic brain injury? What if it happens repeatedly? In these cases, reality testing is our good friend. Listen to what your gut says, but also describe the situation to someone who is completely removed from the situation (perhaps a nurse who works at another facility or a trusted friend) and get their feedback.

Almost every nurse we interviewed said that a very important boundary nurses should maintain is the discipline of leaving work at work. "When you walk out that door," said Kathryn Cantleyan RN, the clinical coordinator of Sarasota Memorial Hospital's Community Medical Clinic, "leave it behind." Some nurses may literally need to leave their work behind, e.g., refuse to bring paperwork home or make work phone calls in off hours. However, most hospital staff nurses don't regularly have the opportunity to flush IVs, give IMs, or do pain assessments on family and friends. For them "leaving work at work" is more about finding a way to decompress after the shift so that thoughts of work are not constantly invading nonworking hours. Many nurses mentioned having a ritual to help smooth the transition from work to home. Don't be put off by the word "ritual." We're not suggesting you need to light enough candles to illuminate your entire metro area or work so hard at twisting yourself into some advanced yoga position that you dislocate a joint or two. Your transition ritual can be something very simple. For some ideas of what other nurses do, see Rituals for Reclaiming the Day.

Maintaining a transition ritual is highly individual and the strength and even complexity of a ritual will vary from person to person and perhaps and from day to day. On days when you are completely beat, you will be tempted to forget about your transition ritual in favor of going right for "zzzzzzz" ritual. Shorten it if possible on these days, but don't abandon it! You may think 'I'm too tired to think about all that work stuff anyway.' But while you may be too tired, your subconscious mind is not. You'll end up processing it in your sleep and having one of those dreams where you find yourself working in an ICU located in the house you lived in as a child, wearing only a flannel shirt and your bunny slippers, and trying to start insert an IV made of black licorice into an uncooperative patient, who seems to be the front desk clerk from the hotel you stayed at one night when you were on vacation 3 years ago. Save yourself the nightmares. Decompress before you sleep.

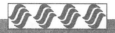

Rituals for Reclaiming the Day

Here is what some nurses suggested:

"I light a candle and think about all the people who love me."

"I imagine myself in a place where I felt really peaceful. For me, this is the beach that I went to with my family as a child. I get all my senses going and really imagine how it smells, sounds, felt to be there. This not only helps me go from work to home mode, but also it imprints this peaceful place on my mind, so when things seem overwhelming (at work or at home), I take a little break and go there!"

"When I get home, I clean a little bit of something…no matter how tired I am! I don't start with anything that will get me worked up (like cleaning out from under the kids' beds!) but something that—with a little effort—I will be able to notice the immediate difference. Doing the dishes (especially by hand) is perfect for this, as well as folding or putting away piled up laundry."

"I write down whatever I am afraid will bug me from now until I go back to work and think is there anything I can do about this? If the answer is yes (for example, if I've forgotten to tell the nurse I signed off to about something) then I immediately do it. If the answer is 'no' I tear the paper up into the tiniest scraps I can and throw it away with a ceremonial flourish."

"I go out with coworkers for coffee or a drink after almost every shift. We give ourselves 7 minutes to vent about the day and then the rule is "no talking about work!" The person who slips and talks about it has to buy the next round."

"I have an old baseball cap I wear on my drive home from work. I let myself ruminate about how unfairly I was treated, how bad the world is, how much I hate nursing or how sad a particular patient's situation is as long as I have the hat on. But only as long as the hat is on do I give myself that permission. So when I park in the driveway, I take off the hat and leave it the car, and tell myself firmly "I'm not wearing the hat, so I choose not to think about it." If I really need to think about something (for example, if I need to problem-solve about working with a particularly difficult patient or doc) I have been known to go out to the car and sit there with my hat on, thinking about what I can do. My family might think I'm a little nutsy but better that than have a preoccupied dad."

(continued)

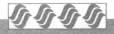

Rituals For Reclaiming the Day *(continued)*

"I have a venting journal which I keep under double lock and key. When I'm feeling pressured from things that have happened at work, I write all my deepest (and yes, very often most unpleasant thoughts) and reactions there. Some of what is reflected there is from external events but I suppose it also lets me get in touch with my 'shadow side...' and really express the selfish, unloving or unprofessional feelings I choose not to act on. I don't re-read it much (reading the profanity I use when upset often shocks me when I'm not in venting mode!) but occasionally I will page through and look for patterns. If there is some situation that I always seem to be venting about, usually I find I need to take some sort of other type of action besides venting!"

"I run away from work! Literally! I live in an apartment about 4 miles from work. If I drove, I would be home in less than five minutes and I would have no down time at all. So I take my running shoes with me, slip them on (scrubs are fine for running in hot weather) and take off. By the time I get home, sometimes I feel so refreshed it's like I never even went to work!"

As for other boundaries, your institution may already provide some policies about your interactions with patients and family members that might guide you. For example, a hospital might make policies about staff members not giving their home phone number to patients (nurses commonly mentioned this as their personal boundary, regardless of hospital policy) or might prohibit staff from accepting gifts from patients or their families, etc. Other boundaries might be very specific to a particular work situation. For example, while it's not commonly considered professional for nurses to eat with their patients, one RN we interviewed works on an eating disorder treatment unit. As part of the therapeutic process, staff members take turns eating their meals in the cafeteria with patients, hoping to model healthy relationships with food. Nurses are told this is a requirement in their initial interview with this unit. A firm boundary of "I don't eat with my patients" wouldn't work well in this case even though it might be a perfectly reasonable limit in another situation.

Of course, patients and families are not the only people with whom nurses have to set boundaries. Nurses also have to set limits with their peers, docs, and others in the workplace. Pay attention to when and where you feel shamed, unreasonably angry, consistently resentful, or downright surly. These are sometimes hints of areas in which we are allowing others to take advantage of us and we might need to set a boundary.

So how do we set these all-important boundaries? *The Nitty Gritty of Boundary Setting* contains, well, obviously the nitty gritty details, but the three overall keys are directness of communication, directness of communication, and oh—did we mention—directness of communication. As unfortunate as it may be, people will not read our minds to find out what is really bugging us when we're grumping around the unit. So the key is to actually tell the person who we feel is taking advantage of us that (get this) we feel they are taking advantage of us and what we would like them to do differently. Also—and we say this with much compassion because we have struggled with this ourselves—grumbling, alas, does not count. The guidelines described in *The Nitty Gritty of Boundary Setting* will work when you need to take the most formal, foolproof route, but most boundaries don't need to be proclaimed with the fanfare of the Academy Awards nominee announcements. You don't even necessarily need to stand up on a chair in the cafeteria and read your new boundary from a parchment scroll or use a hemostat to inscribe it in a marble slab that you place below the scheduling board in the nurses' station. In fact, normal every day boundary setting can be as drama free as saying to a coworker, "Yes, I'd be willing to switch with you for two night shifts this month, but no more." In addition, what we learn about boundary setting in work can be applied to our personal life and vice versa. As Mary Anne Carey, a gerontology nurse with 12 years of experience explains it, "[To develop good boundaries] practice setting limits with self and personal life to be able to set limits with patient care."

One of the most frustrating parts of setting boundaries is that it's not always enough to just tell people what we expect from them, we sometimes have to show them that we mean business. This can be disheartening, especially in a situation where it was difficult to "muster up the gumption" (as Kelli's mom would say) to set the boundary in the first place. Let's say for example, that Nedra Nurse and Nancy Nurse have been working together for some time. They have a reasonably good working relationship, but Nedra Nurse has the annoying habit of bringing a large lunch and taking Nancy Nurse's diet orange soda out of the refrigerator in the break room to make room for the large lunch. After 3 months of drinking warm orange soda, Nancy Nurse catches Nedra Nurse in the break room where Nedra Nurse is heating up coffee and says, "Nedra Nurse, I would appreciate it if you would find some other way to make room in the refrigerator other than moving my drink out." While Nancy Nurse speaks, Nedra Nurse is tapping on the microwave, trying to make it heat the coffee faster. Nedra Nurse responds without

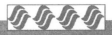

The Nitty Gritty of Setting Boundaries

Setting a boundary can be simple, although it's seldom easy!
One possible recipe:

1. Add an "I statement" followed by a "feeling statement"
   e.g., "I feel angry"
   e.g., "I feel frustrated"
2. To an objective description of the person's behavior (preferably done with out anger in as few words as possible)
   e.g., "when you don't clean up your mess in the break room"
   e.g., "when you put the chart back without telling me you wrote orders on it"
3. Complete with a specific request for changed behavior
   e.g., "So in the future, please don't leave your dirty dishes, for me to clean up."
   e.g., "So from now on, please let me know when you've written orders on one of my patients' charts."

If this sounds like too much (as one nurse said) "pop psychology mumbo-jumbo" to you, you can modify the recipe. The only essential elements are directness in communication and asking for a specific behavior change.
Some more hints:

In certain situations, you might want to omit the feeling statements, for example, when talking about your feelings might be inappropriate or might leave you at a tactical disadvantage.

Remember you can't set a limit and at the same time take care of someone else's feelings.

It might feel weird setting a boundary (you might feel scared or shamed) but that doesn't mean you shouldn't do it!

For best results, follow through on your boundary. If you say "I'm not going to X" and you keep doing X, people will be less likely to believe you when you say, "I'm not going to do Y."

Beware of using "disclaimer words" that weaken your request for changed behavior. Prefacing your request with "I guess," or "I was hoping" or "I was thinking" turns your request into a vague suggestion.

Sometimes patients (and others) are not aware they are asking questions you might consider personal or inappropriate (after all we ask our patients about everything from their sex lives to the last time they moved their bowels). It's helpful to develop stock answers to such questions. They can be gentle redirections (if appropriate for the situation) and still be truthful. For example, "Our facility doesn't allow us to give out our personal phone numbers," or when asked about other personal matters such as how you got a scar, "it's a long story."

looking up from the microwave vigil, "Hmm? Okay. Yeah, I'll try." The next day, do you think Nedra Nurse leaves Nancy Nurse's orange soda in the refrigerator? Nooooooo chance. So for the rest of the week, Nancy Nurse may have to remind Nedra Nurse of the boundary, may have to use different words to explain the boundary or might have to write a note on the refrigerator as a reminder. But if Nancy Nurse cares enough about the boundary and is tenacious in defending it, eventually Nedra Nurse will probably stop taking her orange soda out of the refrigerator. In this case, as in many cases, it's not that Nedra Nurse is against Nancy Nurse, Nedra Nurse is simply for herself.

The same tenacity is sometimes needed when setting boundaries with a patient. As MH, a public health nurse with more than 30 years of experience suggests, "listen to the client/patient's needs. At the same time keep repeating (parroting) the limits." Some additional communication techniques for dealing with boundary transgression can be found in Chapter 6, "Fostering Healthy Relationships."

When you are having difficulty setting or defending a boundary, it can help if you remember that good boundaries are ultimately beneficial for most all those involved. When we don't set boundaries and therefore do things we don't want to do or that are not our responsibility, it usually makes us resentful...big time. In these situations, our work (and ability to work as a part of a team) suffers as a result. When we are able to set boundaries it helps others know what to expect from us, and it makes us happier and even more productive nurses.

Finally, there are some situations in which boundary setting is futile. For example, you can't set a boundary in direct opposition with institutional policy. If your hospital requires mandatory overtime, saying "I'm sorry I cannot work overtime" won't work and could easily get you fired. Even in the absence of an actual policy, it's also difficult to set boundaries in direct opposition to institutional culture. If every other nurse at the managed-care company where you are a case manager comes in at 8 a.m. and works until 7 p.m. four days a week, it's going to be difficult to leave after you've worked 8 hours, even if it is within your rights as an employee to do so. Boundary setting in these two cases is doomed to die an early, perhaps messy, death. In this type of situations, if you feel strongly about your desired boundary, you have two choices: you can work to change institutional policies or culture or you can look for another job. Obvious? Perhaps a little, but as Kathryn Cantley reminded us in the chapter opener, "There are always options, but a lot of nurses can't see them when they're in the midst of it."

For a further discussion of making these types of decisions, see the "When Is It Time to Move On" section, found in Chapter 11.

Do You Smell Smoke? Dealing with Burnout

Like stress, the term "burnout" has become almost a cliché. But when you ask nurses, "What is burnout?" they produce some very vivid definitions:

"When you wake up in the morning, and say 'it's morning already?' "
Karen P Smith, RN

"When it isn't about the patient anymore."
Lourdes Rodriguez, RN

"When you've lost the desire to help people."
ML, RN

"When the nurse truly believes she hates what she does for a living."
Mary Anne Carey, RN

"Not wanting to come to work, being apathetic, not trying, just going through the motions."
MS, RN

"Giving up and having an 'I don't care' attitude, or a negative attitude."
Bob Darrow, RN

"Feelings of anxiety, constant pre-occupation with the job, loss of energy and enthusiasm, misdirected anger, 'I don't care' attitude toward work responsibilities and patients, feelings of dread at the thought of going to work..."
MH, RN

The media is full of images of the burnt-out health care worker; the scary paramedics in the movie *Bringing in the Dead*; Nurse Rachet from *One Flew Over the Cuckoo's Nest* (surely she didn't graduate from nursing school with such a sadistic bedside manner); and the sitcom nurses whose surly manner and nasty comebacks provide fodder for jokes in the "main character gets a tonsillectomy and is accidentally put in the pediatric unit" story line. Away from the silver and small screen, in "real-time" we've all seen nurses who seem to ration pain meds, act as though giving a patient an extra blanket or pillow requires an act of God, and—as one nurse from Wisconsin said, "find fault like they think there's some kind of reward."

But as important as it is to understand what burnout is, we have to understand what it is not. Burnout is not the normal fatigue that results when our generosity of spirit is challenging by the constant demands on it. For example, in the hospital you might find yourself praying that a patient doesn't die on your shift because it's so much extra paperwork. If you work in a clinic, you might role your internal eyes at a patient who states she is finally ready to leave a domestic violence situation, knowing that helping her get into a shelter will blow your chances of getting away early on a lovely Friday afternoon.

We might feel guilty about these feelings, but they are completely normal, and as long as we don't act on them (i.e., provide less than adequate or compassionate care) we should feel no compunction whatsoever. As nurses, we deal with tough stuff day after day after day after day. We are involved in the real muck and sometimes ugliness of life in a way people in few other professions are. Despite the fact that we spend all day, every working day with people who are suffering, at times there is little we can do to lessen their pain. Building up some type of defense against this emotional barrage is normal, even healthy. If we become the nurse version of Sponge Bob Square Pants, soaking up indiscriminately all the pain of life around us, then we'll undoubtedly find ourselves burning out before the ink is dry on our license.

The key to burnout prevention is stress reduction. This chapter includes many techniques for dealing directly with stress in general (including *Nurses' Tips for Stress Management*) but other chapters address the specifics of career challenges that many nurses find stressful. When you create your own *burnout prevention plan* it might be worth your time to take special note of what issues most affect you and review the content of the corresponding chapter. For example, if your biggest work stressor is nurse-to-nurse communication, you might peruse again the chapter on relationships. On the other hand, if nurse-to-nurse communication is not a source of stress for you, but you feel certain practices in your workplace expose nurses to unnecessary liability, you'll want to spend more time with the chapter on legal and ethical concerns.

As we mentioned in Chapter 1, some of the most experienced nurses we talked with urged nurses to begin a process of daily maintenance to sustain their passion for nursing. To do this, you can read biographies of accomplished nurses or other (as one nurse referred to it) "rah rah" literature about nursing, post prominent reminders of why you became a nurse, talk with other nurses who like their jobs, go to professional conventions and even volunteer to work with those wide-eyed, annoyingly enthusiastic nursing students doing their clinical rotations on your floor.

Finally, realize that if you are burned out, it does not have to be a permanent state. SL, RN from Las Cruces, New Mexico, is one nurse who recovered from burnout. "I dropped out for a year [from nursing] and came back. I was a crispy critter after about 15 or so years. I decided that the only people hospital administrators listened to were lawyers. So

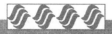

Nurses' Tips for Stress Management

We asked nurses "how do you handle stress?" Here are some of their suggestions:

"Laughter"

Lourdes Rodriguez, RN

"Swimming"

MS, RN

"I work three 12 hour shifts so I spend less time on unit."

GJD, RN

"If I can get away for 5 minutes without putting anyone's life or my job in danger, I go to the bathroom and have a good cry."

TJ, RN

"I try and always keep my perspective. I ask myself 'Is this a problem or just an annoyance?' If it is a genuine problem then I ask myself 'whose problem is it? Can I do anything about it?' Often I find that things that I had assumed responsibility for were things that I had very little control over."

Sarah Thompson, RN

"I take control of something, anything, no matter how little. I use this at work when my day is falling apart. Okay, what do I have to do to keep patient A safe, then patient B and so on. Then, I work my way up Maslow's hierarchy of needs. On three code days, I just have to realize I'm not going to meet everyone's desire for self actualization and have all the patients holding hands and singing kumbaya by the end of the shift. I use this for myself too...what do I have to do to be safe this shift...i.e. ask for help, etc."

PT, RN

"I talk to myself to turn negative thoughts around. Some days I even talk to myself out loud, when I'm in the med room, gathering my meds. I'll have a quiet little monologue going. I talk to myself like I would a friend...'okay honey, it's only 7:30 am, a lot has gone wrong, but the day is not a total loss yet...just get these meds ready and then you can go on to the next thing. If you remember something you need to do, just jot it down....you're doing fine...you're a good nurse and you're doing the best you can for your patients...' It may look a little eccentric to my co-workers but I've worked at this hospital a long time and have a repu-tation as fair person and a hard worker so people tolerate my little self pep talks. A new nurse might have to do them internally."

CS, RN

"Lots of time playing: hot tubs, candy, reading, leaving it...at work. I have my family, my garden my dogs and cats and friends, etc. I can find lots of things to do that do not involve my job."

Regina Moore, RN

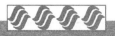

What factor in my job is most stressful to me right now?

Whose problem is this factor? Is there any way to decrease the stress in this area? What would I need to do to change it? Am I willing to do this? What resources do I have now that could help me make the change?

What factor in my life most contributes to job stress? Is there any way I can decrease the stress of this factor? What would it require for me to change it? Am I willing to do this? What resources do I have now that could help me make the change?

What stress management strategies am I currently using? How well do these work? What new strategies would I like to try?

I went to law school. Egad and zounds! After a year I was pretty sure that I had brain damage. [I] could not keep doing anything I hated that much. I came back to nursing (at the same hospital) and realized I loved it. [I've] been back since '91. I finish my MSN in a couple more weeks. I guess I'll keep doing it for a while."

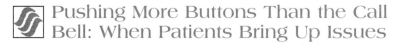

Pushing More Buttons Than the Call Bell: When Patients Bring Up Issues

"It does not do to leave a live dragon out of your calculations if you live near him."

JRR Tolkien

Okay, Tolkien was probably talking about a real live dragon, not a metaphorical one, but we've lifted his quote to start our discussion about unresolved issues because we think the metaphor of the "elephant in the living room" that no one talks about has gotten a little tired with overuse. At any rate, let's get real: very seldom do people become a nurse because they've spent their entire life in relative tranquility and financial security, surrounded by a supportive loving Walton-esque family, picking daisies. For many people, the compassion that nursing requires was developed during long years of serving detention at the school of hard knocks.

So it's not surprising that when we deal with patients or certain situations we are occasionally reminded of someone or something that caused us difficulty in the past, i.e., our own "live dragon living near us." This makes it challenging—but not impossible—to deal with the patient or situation in a professional and objective manner.

Sometimes it's hard to tell if you are reacting to the past rather than the present. For example, most nurses find it challenging to work with patients who seem to be manipulative, or who try to pit staff members against each other (e.g., "Nurse B, I think you're the best nurse here. Nurse A doesn't think so—something about you always giving meds late—but I always stick up for you."). This kind of behavior can make a nurse want to pull out their hair in handfuls, slam their head repeatedly against a wall and/or leave the unit screaming and not stop running until they have crossed the state line. Does this mean this nurse is "getting her buttons pushed" for example, because of some childhood trauma? Not necessarily. Some behavior is simply inherently annoying, and almost anyone would become frustrated with such an exchange. And even if one nurse has a reaction to a situation that is dissimilar to her coworkers, this does not necessarily reflect a "button-pushing" situation. The different reactions may be a result of differences in temperament. For example, one nurse may feel quite irritated when the perfect schedule she has planned is sidelined with a new admission that appears on the floor with no notice. Another nurse might welcome the novelty of the interruption and enjoy taking a break from her planned tasks.

Of the nurses we interviewed, most said they had at least one patient in their career who really pushed their buttons. MH, a nurse with more than 20 years of experience said, "[When a patient is pushing my buttons] I don't always know initially but then I find myself feeling at a loss for words, then I might tend to become dismissive or feel very nervous and lacking in confidence." In other examples, one nurse said she struggled to give good care to alcoholics because her father was an alcoholic who abused her as a child. And patients aren't the only ones that can remind us of something we'd rather forget. Other nurses, docs, the housekeeping staff, even the smell of the spinach surprise in the cafeteria are all potential triggers for reliving painful past experiences.

If you find yourself saying, "I don't understand why I'm so upset about this" and you are not tired, hungry, or otherwise stressed, the issue might very well be about the past rather than the present. It's important to note that the situation doesn't have to be exactly the same as a situation in the past to cause a reaction. It only has to remind you of it in some way (possibly on a subconscious level) so that you are stimulated to react in a way you might not typically react. Or as one nurse said, "If I'm crying about a tough situation when I would normally be laughing it off, it's not about the patient, it's about me."

When we respond not to the present but to the past, the results can be less than fun and may be downright scary. But what do we do about it?

First, identify the nature of the problem. In some cases, the situation may be making you so miserable that you'll have figured out there is some kind of problem yourself. Or a trusted coworker may let you know if you seem to be irrationally annoyed with a particular patient or situation, or might mention that it seems you are letting professional boundaries slip. Also, your family members will definitely let you know if you are coming home consistently and inordinately crabby. Just figuring out you are getting your buttons pushed gets you out of the past and into the present a bit.

Knowing you are getting your buttons pushed also gives you a sense of control. You can stop berating yourself for your feelings and concentrate on the next step. "[When I find a patient is pushing my buttons] I try to immediately recognize this and control spontaneous responses," said Molly Raimondi, a Pennsylvania RN with 31 years of experience as a nurse. Relatively new grad Jill Hall adds that in this situation, "I grit my teeth and try and stay professional."

The response of one Colorado nurse outlined one of the most important next steps, getting support, "[when getting my buttons pushed] I try to recognize that this is happening and breathe through it…afterwards I will discuss my feelings with a trusted friend and process." If you've not used the buddy system since swimming at summer camp in eight grade, dig it out of the mothballs now. For example, if you are dealing with a surgeon whose yelling reminds you of your Aunt Mildred who traumatized you with her screaming as a child, ask another nurse to be around the nurses' station when you ask the surgeon—one more time—to not leave sharps in the patient's bed after completing a bedside procedure. You don't necessarily need to detail the whole Aunt Mildred 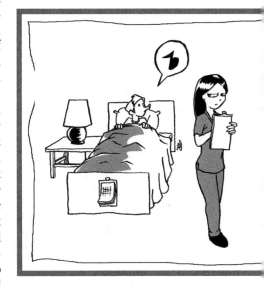 connection to your buddy nurse and explain that you don't need assistance with an intervention (unless you do), just a supportive presence.

In certain short-term situations, most nurses reported they were generally able to manage their reaction by limiting their exposure to it, usually by trading assignments with another nurse. Bob Darrow, a nurse of 28 years, explained, "[When a patient really pushes my buttons] I respectfully leave after I give their care. I also inform the charge nurse regarding this issue, for a possible future change in assignment."

Nurses acknowledged that finding a long-term solution for recurring button-pushing situations could be tricky. For example, if a nurse's father died of lung cancer, and the nurse works on an oncology floor, it wouldn't be practical for the nurse to be assigned only young or female patients because every cachectic older male who chomps on a cigar and demands to be taken down for a smoke break reminds the nurse of a father's protracted illness.

In these situations, the twin tools of *grounding statements and self soothing* can be quite helpful in controlling reactions.

There may be a time when you find that despite having tons of support, making grounding statements until your face turns purple and self-soothing up a storm, you still are not able to deal with a certain type of patient or work situation. In this case, it might be worth a visit (or a few visits) to your friendly neighborhood mental health professional.

Grounding and Self-Soothing

Grounding and self-soothing are twin remedies for when you're getting your buttons pushed.

Grounding is a way of settling yourself more firmly in the present. It helps you act, rather than react, when confronted with triggering situations. Examples of grounding actions include:

- Positive, present-oriented self-talk (e.g., "I'm feeling like a kid in this situation but I know I am really an adult and a capable professional. I can handle this situation")
- Focusing on your present actions (e.g., feeling yourself walk to the water fountain, get a drink, concentrating on how the water feels in your mouth, how your feet feel on the floor, etc.)

The pesky thing about being "grounded" is that instead of being lost in your reaction, you have to feel all your feelings (is this starting to sound like something developed by the Stuart Smalley character on *Saturday Night Live*?). This is almost never fun.

In order to keep your emotions from galloping out of control, it's helpful to use self-soothing techniques that calm you through their effects on one of your five senses. For example, depending on the situation you might squeeze a stress ball, listen to music, sneak a 30-second glance at a picture you have taped to your clipboard of a beautiful Caribbean beach, or let a piece of hard candy dissolve on your tongue.

This requires a commitment of time and money, but it's not only an investment in your career, it's an investment in your personal growth. You may come out the other side feeling a small bit of thankfulness that your nursing experiences forced you to deal with a ghost from your past, because as Florida RN Kathryn Cantley said, "If you can recognize that you're having your buttons pushed and deal with it in a healthy productive way, that's called evolution."

Physical Stressors and Occupational Hazards

The nurses we interviewed for this book associated a number of physical problems with work as a nurse. Some of the risks for these maladies can only be addressed on a facility-wide level. For example, bladder problems and back injuries may be decreased by providing adequate staffing so that nurses aren't forced to go an entire shift without using the bathroom, or lift without needed assistance. Nurses can use their collective bargaining units or organize in other ways to put pressure on administrators to work toward a safer working environment.

Given the limits of administrative responsiveness, it makes sense for nurses to also do what they can to prevent on the job injuries, and the nurses we interviewed had plenty of suggestions for how to do that. Mostly their suggestions emphasized paying close attention to the basics we learned as students, in fact, putting together their comments resulted in a piece of text that might easily be called "Everything I Need to Know About Preventing Injuries I Learned in Nursing School":

"Wear support hose. Go to the bathroom when you feel the urge, instead of holding it for hours. Take breaks even if you don't smoke."

DL, RN, 23 years' experience

"[Get] appropriate help, don't believe that all tasks can be completed alone."

Mary Anne Carey, RN

"Stay in shape, take good care of yourself. " MS, RN
"Don't work more than two 12 hour shifts in a row, drink enough water during the shift."

Jill Hall, RN, new grad in California

Other nurses added:

"Deal with sleep disturbances early and aggressively;"

"Exercise to avoid weight gain. Our job is so physical, even a small gain makes things so much more difficult!"

"Don't try and save time by rushing when you're around sharps. HIV, Hepatitis C are the gifts that keep on giving!"

"Use good body mechanics and always, always, always get help when lifting"

Regina Moore summed up the responses of many nurses, "I do not think these physical maladies can be avoided. You are on your feet all the time, moving lifting [dealing with] violent patients, etc. I say be as careful as you can all the time and take time to heal the healer."

To find additional information on preventing and dealing with specific physical stressors and occupational hazards of nursing, see the Resources section of this chapter.

Humor as a Stress Modulator

Okay, we admit we are almost obsessed with this subject, in fact, in the um...prequel to this book, *How to Survive and Maybe Even Love Nursing School*, we devoted an entire appendix to a discussion of using humor for healing. We won't repeat the content offered there, but we do want to reinforce—it's okay to laugh at work! We feel this is important to mention not because we feel nurses don't display a sense of humor. Instead we've found that most nurses seem to have a natural ability to find the funny in very difficult situations, but many nurses seem to feel vaguely ashamed of our propensity for "gallows humor," perhaps thinking it is disrespectful of patients.

Certainly we don't want patients and families to overhear the kind of joking nurses do to let off steam, but if you have a break room with a closed door or other private place, go for it! With all the ever-growing evidence that laughter decreases stress, increases endorphin levels, and aids in immune response, (check out some of the resources listed at the end of this chapter for specifics), perhaps hospital administrators will start requiring each nurse to share a specified number of wisecracks about body fluids per shift. Until that moment, though, don't be afraid to enjoy each other and make each other laugh!

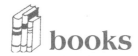 books

Elkin, Allen (1999).
Stress Management for Dummies. Hoboken, NJ: IDG Books.

Oy, again with the word "dummies" in the title, but we're recommending this book anyway, because it can give you tons and tons of ideas for reducing stress in your life. An additional lovely feature is the appendix, which provides step-by-step instructions on how to make your own guided relaxation tape.

Ellis, Albert (1999).
How to Make Yourself Happy and Remarkably Less Disturbable. Atascadero, CA: Impact Publishers.

Okay, the Microsoft Word spellchecker insists that "disturbable" is not a word, but that doesn't distract from the usefulness of this book. Written from a rational emotive therapy point-of-view, readers can use the suggestions provided to help reduce the stress of tasks left undone or procrastination. In fact, just checking out the whimsical cover illustrations ought to make you happy and a tad less stressed, for a moment at least.

Passoff, Michelle (1998).
Lighten Up: Free Yourself from Clutter. New York, NY: Perennial Press.

The subtitle of this book is "create the space for miracles by freeing yourself from too much stuff," which sounds like a worthy—if lofty— goal to us. Yup, stress equals clutter, no two ways about it. This is a practical guide to what you need to keep and what you can throw away. Good for those of us who have been on the planet a while and have amassed way too many little scraps of paper and also may be useful for the traditional age new grad who wishes to avoid creating a paper-clutter monster.

Smith, Manuel J (1985).
When I Say No, I Feel Guilty. New York: NY, Bantam Books.

Ah, the oft-sighed statement of nurses everywhere! This classic of assertiveness training is as relevant today as it was when it was released nearly two decades ago. The book was recently updated. Worth taking a gander, if just to read through some of the many role-playing scenarios you can learn from.

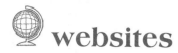 websites

The Center for Disease Control's Stress at Work Report
www.cdc.gov/niosh/stresswk.html
This report is not specific to nursing workplace stress but it's relevant because it provides research-based documentation that stress does affect the bottom line. Also details what changes need to be made in workplaces in order to reduce the amount of stress workers face. The report is in the public domain so you can reprint articles for sharing with coworkers, surreptitiously leaving on your nurse manager's desk, etc.

Nurse Care
www.care-nurse.com
Nurse-Care, appropriately sub-titled "Caring for the Nurse," includes lots of inspirational articles, nurses' prayers, creeds, etc., and also some real-life nursing humor. Includes pics of diploma program uniforms from the olden days and a list of duties for nurses in the 1800s, making us extremely grateful for the state of modern nursing.

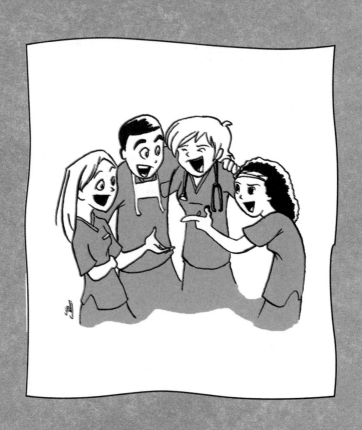

CHAPTER

The Long and Winding Road: Don't Forget About Your Future

A Nurse Speaks

"I wouldn't say I'm afraid of the future...for me as a nurse, or for nursing as a profession. But I can see the signs of the times; I'm worried about what this shortage is going to do to working conditions, and I'm thinking about what that will mean for me. So am I worried? No, but I'm planning."

Beth Drummond, RN

 Reviewing Your Career Ladder Goals

S o here we are. You've found a job, a mentor, and a support system. You've survived job interviews, shift work, your first week—maybe your first month, first year, or first decade—as a nurse. We've chatted about stress management, time management, and dealing with the management. What's next?

Well, before we even get started in this discussion we want to make it 100%, perfectly, absolutely, abundantly crystal clear that when we say "career ladder goals" we are NOT suggesting that climbing a "career ladder" is all about getting an advanced degree, or a certain level of experience so that you can leave bedside nursing. This kind of presumption (sometimes found in some of the more traditional career guides and journals) implies that being a staff nurse is mostly a stepping stone to something bigger, better, and possibly more lucrative. This is not the case for most of the nurses we interviewed. In fact, many nurses said they would not consider any type of nursing position that didn't involve direct patient care, because, as one North Caroline nurse with more than 25 years of experience explained, "I wouldn't put up with the craziness that is health care today except for one reason: to make the difference in a life of a patient. Anything else—even if it was good, helpful work—would not satisfy me."

So, when we talk of "career ladder" we mean a ladder of your own design, leading where you want to go in nursing, which may or may not lead to more power, prestige, or money. Okay? Enough said.

You've probably already started thinking ahead to your "career ladder" goals, even if you are quite happy (for now) in your current position. Maybe you had wild, dreamy thoughts since nursing school— or maybe even long before—about what kind of nurse you'd ideally like to be, what kind of patient population you'd ideally like to work with, or where you'd ideally like to practice. One nurse we talked with had always wanted to be an interoperative photographer (who knew there was such a thing?), another wanted to do travel nursing in Hawaii.

Or maybe your dreams were about developing a working life that would enable you to achieve a non–work-related goal. For example, one nurse might want to work part-time so she has more time for training her Iditarod-hopeful French poodle sled-dog team, another nurse might want to work nights so he can be there for his kids when they come home after school.

When you were just getting your feet (proverbially) wet, dealing with new grad exhaustion, learning to juggle more patients, and begging back into the good graces of family members who felt neglected while you were in school, perhaps these dreams seemed unrealistic to you. Now is the time to bring them back to the (once again, proverbial) front burner and see what kind of (proverbial) recipe you can put together to bring your dreams to a (proverbial) boil without getting (metaphorically speaking) burned. In other words, it's time to plan!

Since you've gotten through school, gotten your license and at least your first job, you clearly have the ability to set goals and develop the plans to meet those goals. Therefore, we will not bore with you several thousand pages of goal-setting theories (this as much for us as it for you; the publisher tends to get a little testy when we turn in a manuscript that's several thousand pages over the page limit), but we would like to remind you of a few quick goal-setting hints.

First, (we know you remember this from nursing school) goals have to be measurable and specific. Much to our frustration, our clinical instructors never let us get away with writing "Mr. Smith will have a much better day today than he did yesterday" in the goal part of the care plan. We bet your clinical instructors didn't either. So when you formulate your goal, make sure it contains specifics. "I will get my MSN with a 3.8 GPA" is much easier to work toward than "I will continue to learn as a nurse."

Second, goals need to have target completion dates. Human beings have an amazing capacity for procrastination. In fact, when we were nearing the deadline for getting this chapter done, we began to think "hmm...is this a unique characteristic of humans or do other animals procrastinate?" So, of course, we really needed to do some research about animals and procrastination and we couldn't find the information we needed on the Internet. So we ended up doing some field observations and found that—as far as we could see—it appears other animals do not procrastinate. It was however, difficult to decide exactly what they would be procrastinating about, if they were, in fact, procrastinating. Anyway, we had a lovely day at the zoo. Which brings us to our next point, which is the human capacity for rationalization is amazing, but the human capacity for rationalization about our procrastination is even more striking. That's why we need deadlines or things don't get done.

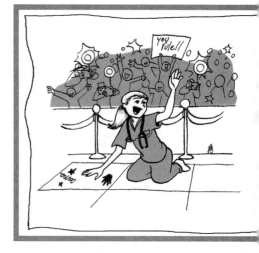

Third, share your goals. Selectivity is the key to making this tip work. It's best to share with someone who can hold you accountable without being a complete pest.

One last thing about career ladder planning—don't be discouraged if the path to your goals seems to be a nonlinear one. First of all, life circumstances change. A nurse who is a single mother with two school-aged children might have the goal to become a diabetes educator and be working toward her certification. This might be possible with her children as her main outside responsibility, but if the nurse's mother becomes ill and has to live with the nurse and her family, the diabetes educator plan might have to go on hold for a while. Being "on hold" is not the same as abandoned, and it might be that the nurse can find another, less time-consuming way to work toward her goal until she can resume classes.

In addition, some of the nurses we spoke with said that their best work experiences were the result of serendipitous events that landed them in a position of working with a patient population they would have never predicted. MP, a Pennsylvania nurse, said her work in pediatrics, home visiting, and long-term care were all "very interesting" but not exactly what she wanted. When she needed some extra cash after the holidays one year, a friend told her about a temporary per diem position in the county prison. From the first day, MP said, "I fell in love with correctional nursing. I feel it uses all my skills and all my talents. I enjoy interacting with the staff and my patients and crafting a balance between being both tough and being compassionate as the situation dictates."

Although many of the nurses we talked with were making some plans for the future, they emphasized that the flexibility of nursing and the diversity of nursing made it possible for them to keep their options open. "I see my career as an ongoing flow through the remainder of my life," said Kathryn Cantley, a clinical coordinator who has worked 19 years as a nurse. "I'm still going to school at age 52, and my guess is that I'll use all my skills later in life to volunteer in the medical field as a nurse."

Lifelong Learning: Academic and Continuing Education Options

Of course, when we think about meeting long-term career objectives we have to consider, at least, the possibility of going back to school. If you're still in the throes of post-traumatic stress disorder from the process of getting your RN, you might take comfort in the fact that most nurses we talked with who were involved in post RN study found it to be a completely different experience than what went on during their pre-licensed days.

"The difference is pretty clear," said one nurse who is currently in an RN to MSN program, "the instructors treat us like we have a brain in our heads." Not that simply being treated "as if you have a brain in your head" is everything a satisfactory experience is made of, but it is a nice place to start.

Many of the nurses we talked with were pursuing an academic nursing degree, with the most common goal being a BSN. The vast majority of nurses were provided tuition reimbursement or tuition assistance as part of the benefits of their jobs and many described this as the main push for getting their BSN. "I'm not going to get much more money if I get my BSN, at least not here," said one new RN who was in his first year working at a long-term care facility, "but as long as it's paid for I'm going. I'm staying here for now, but I'd suggest every nurse get their BSN. You might need it to pursue other opportunities later." We couldn't have said it better ourselves!

Some of the nurses we talked with were pursuing advanced academic degrees, mostly in MSN programs leading to the clinical positions of nurse practitioner or clinical nurse specialist. A much smaller number were involved in MSN programs with a nonclinical track, for example, programs leading to specialization in nursing administration.

Of the nurses not pursuing post-BSN degrees, most were simply not interested in the role that an advanced degree would lead to, fearing that it would be too limiting in scope of practice. One ICU nurse who recently completed a family nurse practitioner program, plans to continue her work as a RN. "I finished the program because I like to finish what I start," she explained, "but I have no intention of working as a nurse practitioner. Many of my classmates are thrilled with their new role and I'm happy for them. But I prefer assessing to diagnosing. I really am a floor nurse at heart. I guess I had only a vague idea of what NPs do when I started. I would suggest to anyone going for one of the advanced nursing degrees to spend a day with an NP or a CNS or whatever and really see what they do on a day-to-day basis."

Many nurses said they were interested in pursuing an advanced degree but felt trapped between financial and time limitations. As one nurse explained, "I can't afford financially to go to school without tuition reimbursement, which I only get if I work full time. But if I work full-time there is no way I can go to school, not without leaving my children unsupervised for long periods of time. If it's a choice between school and letting my kids roam the streets...c'mon, what would you pick?"

However, there are ways around this full-time work meaning no time for school dilemma. First of all, while it's not yet common, some institutions are now offering tuition reimbursement (sometimes at reduced rates) for part-time nurses. If you are interested in going back to school at some point, the availability of tuition reimbursement for part-time nurses may be something to weigh when considering job offers. In addition, because of the nursing shortage, there are burgeoning scholarship opportunities available, many of which will pay for post-RN education. The Johnson and Johnson–sponsored Website www.discovernursing. com lists many of these scholarships and will even match you with a school that meets the eligibility criteria. Finally, if you can borrow the money for school, either through a private lender or a federal student loan program you may become eligible for loan forgiveness (through federal or state entities) if you work in an underserved area after graduation. More information about loan forgiveness programs is available through some of the Websites listed in the Resource section of this chapter.

It is worth a special note that for nurses interested in becoming nurse educators, there are many new scholarship opportunities and loan forgiveness programs that have been developed in the last few years.

More information about these programs can be found through—oh you guessed it—the Websites listed in the Resources section of this chapter.

Although not all nurses we talked with were pursuing academic degrees, all were engaged in some sort of continuing education. For some, the continuing education was in the form of ongoing recertifications required through their employer (e.g., BCLS, ACLS), while others attended conferences and others earned their CE credits by reading journal articles and taking CE tests, either written or online.

If you are struggling to obtain CEs, there are some tricks to make it easier. First, if you can get your employer to pay for you to attend a conference in your specialty area, it can be a less painful way to learn, especially if it's an out of town conference where you're away from your daily life's hassles and can really concentrate on the subject matter. A conference is also a great place to meet other nurses with similar interests, maybe even find a mentor, and attend some very fun toga parties (okay, maybe those were just the conferences we went to).

If you are computer savvy (you are computer savvy, right?) you can also obtain continuing education online. Some state nurses' associations offer online CE free to their members. Other online continuing education is available through commercial sources, such as nursing career guides and CE-specific sites. Some even allow you to obtain your test results immediately and print your own certificates. Before doing your CE requirements online however, check with your state board of nursing about relevant stipulations. Some states, such as Texas, require a certain percentage of continuing education credit to come from live, in-person (not just real-time!) classes.

Changing Issues in Nursing (and How to Make a Change)

Although we've been talking about current issues in nursing throughout this book, we wanted to take a little time in this wrap-up chapter to, well, wrap-up all we've been saying about the different issues and challenges facing our profession today.

Which means we need to talk about, yup, you guessed it, the nursing shortage. If you're like us and many of the nurses we talked with, you may be getting mighty exhausted by all the constant attention focused on the shortage as well as the (sometimes) unspoken pressure for nurses to "do something about it."

One NICU nurse from New York said, "[I went to a nursing convention and] all the speakers talked about the nursing shortage and our responsibility. It reminded me of school on the day before a long holiday. The teacher would look around at all the empty desks and say 'where is everybody? Why are so many students absent?' and I'd always think 'I don't know. But I know I'm here!' "

With this kind of bombardment it's easy to become apathetic. At the same time, the situation—no matter how you look at it—is serious. According to U.S. Bureau of Labor Statistics (the federal agency we trust to keep tabs on things like this for us) more than 1 million new and replacement nurses will be needed by 2010 (Bureau of Labor Statistics, 2001). One million. That bypasses "serious" and goes straight into the heart of the "scary" realm. Thinking about how this will affect patient care, our daily working lives, and the health-care system in general is the stuff that nightmares are made of.

So, what can we do about it? Well, according to the American Association of Colleges of Nursing* the major causes for the nursing shortage are:

1. A shortage of nursing school faculty is restricting nursing program enrollments.
2. With fewer new nurses entering the profession, the average age of the RN is climbing.
3. The total population of registered nurses is growing at the slowest rate in 20 years.
4. Changing demographics signal a need for more nurses to care for our aging population.
5. Job burnout and dissatisfaction are driving nurses to leave the profession.

A quick peruse of these factors reveals that there are some issues contributing to the nursing shortage that as individuals, we can do nothing about. For example, unless one of us has an inside scoop on the current whereabouts of Ponce de Leon, No. 4 is pretty much out of our control. If we have the desire to get an additional academic degree or two and become a nurse educator, we might be able to do our little part to mitigate the nursing faculty shortage.

The rest of the factors pretty much detail the more obvious causes of the nursing shortage—too few people are becoming nurses and too many nurses are leaving the nursing profession.

Since the same number of employers is competing for fewer RNs, employers are scrambling—big time—to compete for the nurses who are out there. You only need to open up a nursing career magazine to the classifieds to see the biggest carrot they're dangling—money, often in the

*   Source: American Association of Colleges of Nursing, 2003.

form of sign-on bonuses. Various government entities are offering similar financial carrots, usually loan forgiveness and repayment plans in
exchange for a certain period of service in a high-need area.

We say "hip, hip hurray" for money, "hip, hip hurray" for sign-on
bonuses, "hip, hip hurray" for nurses finally getting paid (closer) to what
they're worth. But, as Staci's Uncle Morris has been known to say, "It
ain't all about the money, honey."

In fact, if there are any possible positive outcomes of the nursing
shortage they will not be primarily about increased nurse salaries. The
best possible outcome would be that the health-care industry will have
to look closely at the conditions that have been created that make nurses
want to leave bedside nursing. Nonsense such as assigning nurses unrealistic (and dangerous) patient loads, requiring nurses to supervise unlicensed (and untrained) assistive personnel who have taken on nursing
responsibilities, and requiring mandatory overtime and floating will not
seem like such brilliant cost-cutting measures when institutions cannot
find nurses to work for them no matter how huge the sign-on bonus
they offer.

This is where our actions can have an impact on not only the nursing
shortage, but the health-care industry as a whole. We can advocate for
the nursing profession on the micro level, by promoting nursing within
our workplace and our area of personal influence; suggestions on how
to do this can be found in The Art of Advocating for Nursing. We can
also advocate on the macro level through involvement in politics (e.g.,
lobbying for patient-nurse ratio legislation), promoting nursing in the
media, and participation in nursing advocacy groups (collective bargaining organizations, state nurses' associations, etc.).

In addition, we can use our positions as sought-after health-care
professionals to push our employers to provide working conditions that
contribute to a less stressful working environment. The list of favorable
working conditions developed by the National Institute for Occupational
Safety and Health might be a good place to start.

Hopefully, advocating for all these changes will help us feel more
confident about the possibilities of our profession and make us more
likely to suggest it as a profession to people we actually like. Some very
interesting tips on how to do personal recruiting (especially with young
people) can be found in Talk with Kids About Nursing! And if you're
really gung ho about personally recruiting all 1 million nurses we'll be
needing in the next decade or so, check out some of the nursing promotion resources described at the end of this chapter. They can hook you
up with organizations in your area that will be glad to lasso some of that
recruitment energy.

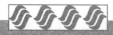

The Art of Advocating for Nursing

- Make sure your patients know you are a registered nurse.
- Fight to keep credentials on ID badges. When unlicensed assistive person-nel have simply "nursing" on their ID, the general public usually does not understand this is a department rather than a title.
- Never use the phrase "just a nurse," even sarcastically.
- In social situations, when people ask you about your occupation, say "I'm a nurse," and spend time explaining what you really do (be careful about how much graphic detail you share at dinner parties!)
- Whether or not you have children, offer to be a guest speaker at a local school. You can come for career day, or offer to be a guest lecturer about some aspect of science or health care.
- Offer to help with tours of your workplace, "bring-your-kid-to-work" type programs and anything else that helps the public be exposed to what nurses do.

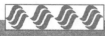

Promoting Nursing in the Media

The media is full of inaccurate and insulting images of nurses and the nursing profession. We can hold media outlets accountable for their actions and present a more positive alternative.

- Write letters of correction and protest whenever you see media images of nursing that are inaccurate. These might be found in newspapers, maga-zines, on TV, films or in advertisements. Send copies to other nurses you know as well as your state nurses' association, to encourage others to share their views.
- When you see an accurate presentation of nurses in the media, write a letter of commendation.
- Become a member of a nursing advocacy organization that monitors media presentations of nurses (e.g., www. nursingadvocacy.com). Sign up for e-mail alerts so that the organization can let you know when a rapid public response to a particular media portrayal of nursing is needed.
- Write letters to the editor about important health-care topics. Identify your-self as a nurse.
- Contact the public interest section of your local newspaper to suggest ideas for stories that focus on the contributions of nursing. If you don't have any luck with your daily paper, contact one of the alternative newspapers (usually published on a weekly basis in most large cities.)

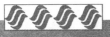

What Makes a Work Environment Less Stressful?

According to the National Institute for Occupational Safety and Health (NIOSH), the federal agency responsible for conducting research and making recommendations for the prevention of work-related injuries, the following factors decrease the amount of stress workers experience on the job:

- Ensuring that the workload is in line with workers' capabilities and resources.
- Designing jobs to provide meaning, stimulation, and opportunities for workers to use their skills.
- Clearly defining workers' roles and responsibilities.
- Giving workers opportunities to participate in decisions and actions affecting their jobs.
- Improving communications reduces uncertainty about career development and future employment prospects.
- Providing opportunities for social interaction among workers.
- Establishing work schedules that are compatible with demands and responsibilities outside the job.

Source: From the National Institute for Occupational Safety and Health's report on Stress at Work (http://www.cdc.gov/niosh/stresswk.html).

Financial Goals and Retirement Strategies

We encountered an interesting phenomenon when we compiled the written surveys that nurses filled out for this book. When we asked, "Are you satisfied with your current retirement plans?" most of the more experienced nurses wrote "no" in capital letters, followed by many exclamation points. This may not be particularly surprising, because an older nurse would presumably be closer to retirement and therefore thinking more about it. However, these responses contrasted even more sharply than you might think with the responses of the younger nurses, who almost without exception left the question blank or replied with multiple question marks.

Perhaps this is why older nurses agreed on one piece of advice about financial planning—do it! For example, one older nurse said, "Start saving as soon as you start working;" another nurse said, "Save early and consistently," and another nurse added, "I wish I had actually started to save with my very first job. I would be amazingly rich today!"

Saving, of course, is a good start, especially for new grads. Celeste Carnage, an ED nurse and death investigator suggested, "New young

Talk with Kids about Nursing!

By Dennis R. Sherrod, EdD, RN

The North Carolina Center for Nursing is replicating a study conducted in the United Kingdom by holding focus group discussions with sixth, 10th and 12th graders to determine their perceptions of nursing careers. Based on a 1998 Foskett & Hemsley-Brown study, funded by the North Carolina Center for Nursing through a Robert Wood Johnson Colleagues in Caring grant, findings from nursing literature and current discussions with youth, we are making a number of suggestions to individuals who talk with young people about nursing.[5]

Predominantly, young people who have selected nursing as a career either have a nurse in their family or otherwise developed a relationship with a nurse.[5,6] For most it is a family member, such as an aunt, but for others it may be a nurse they have close contact with. For example, one student stated she wanted to become a nurse because she was influenced by a nurse who was the mom of a child for whom she provided babysitting services.

As we talk with kids about nursing we need to **make them aware of the intellectual challenge and high level of knowledge nursing involves**.[5,7] The young kids we talked with look forward to participating in a career that requires critical thinking and continued learning. They understand they must meet challenging entry standards for worthwhile careers.

Talk about nurses as autonomous practitioners.[5,7] Inform young people of the many independent decisions that nurses make on a moment-by-moment basis. Essentially, the public's perception continues to be that nurses "take physician's orders" or "assist physicians." People need to know that today's nurse is a collaborative member of the health-care delivery team.

Discuss the variety of work available at all levels.[5,6] Nurses work in a wide array of organizations, such as hospitals, schools, health departments, industries, schools of nursing, home health agencies, law offices, etc. They have the opportunity to work with multiple age groups from neonates to geriatrics. And there are a variety of specialty areas, such as emergency care, critical care, labor and delivery, pediatrics, etc. Let kids know that their interests may change throughout their career and nursing provides a wide variety of work options.

Inform them of the opportunities for career progression.[5] Let them know about options of working as a staff nurse, supervisor, nurse manager, etc. Tell them we see nurses moving into chief executive officer positions in health-care systems since nurses hold a keen understanding of quality patient care and health care delivery.

(continued)

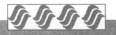

Talk with Kids about Nursing! *(continued)*

Explain the wide range of career opportunities within nursing.[5] Nursing offers an interesting choice of careers since you may enter at a number of levels. Some may begin as a nursing assistant. Others begin as a licensed practical nurse or registered nurse. Even as a registered nurse you may enter with a diploma, associate or baccalaureate education level. Of course, with additional education, registered nurses may move into advanced practice registered nurse positions, such as a nurse practitioner, certified registered nurse anesthetist, clinical specialist, or nurse midwife. Nurses may also work as lawyers, educators, and nurse researchers.

Talk about the idea of "helping people" or "making a difference."[5,6,8] Almost unanimously students state they are interested in nursing because they want to "help people" or "make a difference." So help them understand how nurses help people on a daily basis and how you make a difference in the lives of the people in your community.

Avoid the "Squeamish Factor."[5,6] The most frequent reported reasons for not being interested in nursing are blood, death, fear of giving injections, etc. We need to be very sensitive about how we discuss these subject areas. If these subjects come up they need to be approached softly, depending on the sensitivity of the student.

As we talk with youth, we need to inform them of the need to prepare themselves academically to enter nursing programs. They need to know that today's nursing requires bright, intelligent individuals. Recommend they focus particularly on science and mathematics. Give them examples of how your nursing role uses this knowledge on a regular basis.

Seek out opportunities to speak to students or community groups. Presentations on nursing are an excellent recruitment strategy.[9] Another strategy is to arrange a "Shadow a Nurse" experience, which allows students to have a personal experience with nurses in actual work situations, including carefully guided shadow experiences in different departments.[9,10]

nurses out of school should put 20–25% of their pay aside. When you are not used to making a lot of money you won't miss it. And the more you make the more you'll spend." Many nurses expressed similar thoughts.

In addition to starting to save early, some nurses mentioned that avoiding credit card debt was crucial to being able to meet their financial goals. Although this is much more easily talked about than done, one nurse had this tip, "When I think about using my credit card to pay for something, I think about how much the interest will cost me, not in terms of dollars, but in terms of hours worked, especially if I won't be able to pay off the balance right away. That diamond tennis bracelet stops looking quite so beautiful when I think that I would have to work an entire shift just to pay for the interest if I buy it on credit and only pay the minimum for a few months. If I really want it, I can wait, save and pay cash." Despite these types of efforts, many nurses, like the population in general, are in significant credit card debt. If this is the case for you, you can take advantage of free consumer credit counseling available through nonprofit agencies. There are Websites listed in the Resources section of this chapter that can help you find an agency near you.

If you are frustrated with your spending patterns and can't seem to get your expenses under control, there are several Websites and books listed in the Resource section that may help you. Don't be alarmed by their use of the term "simple living," which for some people conjures up images of dwelling in the woods, wearing clothes made of burlap, eating wild roots and berries, and bathing only once a year. Simple living is not about becoming Grizzly Adams (unless, of course, that's your goal) but about helping us to examine our spending and what we own in terms of "real costs," including the amount of time it takes to maintain our (as Tracy Chapman says) "mountains of things."

So, saving and not spending money you don't have, that seems like pretty basic stuff, right? And you, faithful reader, might be asking "Aren't they going to give some REAL financial planning advice?" Well, actually, no. We're nurses, remember? And since we don't want the average Joe or Jane Accountant or Fred or Flossie Financial Adviser running around starting IVs or assessing lung sounds, in fairness we should stay off their turf. We will, however, pass along some advice that a financial adviser who specializes in working with nurses and other health-care personnel gave to us and add one last thought. If talking or thinking about money and money issues makes you feel sad/strange/weird/angry, don't be too hard on yourself.

Perhaps because nursing has traditionally been a female profession and therefore sometimes provided the second income in a household (e.g., in the case of the so-called "appliance nurses" who went to work when the family needed a new stove or refrigerator), strong personal financial awareness has not always been a part of our professional culture. Starting to think in terms of personal financial goals can be difficult, perhaps making us feel we went into nursing for the wrong reasons. But thinking about taking care of yourself financially in no way detracts from your dedication to patients or to the profession, it only ensures that you can take care of yourself while you are taking care of others. Also, remember, money and how we spend and save it are hard issues for most people in our culture. We have a friend who is now an accountant and has been a psychotherapist. He said that many more clients cry in his office now when talking about their finances than ever cried when talking to him about their phobias or their parents.

An Accountant Speaks: Financial Planning for Nurses

We talked with Walter W. Moyer, accountant and President of The Bottom Line Inc., a Philadelphia-based firm that provides accounting, tax, consulting, and mortgage service that specializes in tax services and financial services for nurses and other health-care professionals.

Q. Let's say a nurse is just starting to think in terms of a financial plan; what are the first things he or she should do?

A. For anyone, no matter what their profession, it's never too late to start financial planning. And you can start pretty simply. The first thing to do is reduce unsecured debt (e.g., car loan, credit cards) have an emergency fund equal to 3 months' living expenses and save either in retirement funds, mutual funds, or money markets.

Q. What should nurses know about minimizing their tax burden?

A. Keep track of every single expense relative to your job. People think of uniforms and shoes and of course a nurse can write off those things, but there are many other deductions that can be claimed. Think about the journals you subscribe to, etc., maybe you buy special pens that you only use for charting. Even a newspaper you buy to read an article that will enhance your nursing skills, that's deductible, and it all adds up.

Q. What should nurses do to optimize their use of "cafeteria" benefit plans available through their employer?

A. The single biggest thing they should do is if the employer provides a matching retirement fund the nurse should put in the maximum amount, especially since it's tax deferred.

Q. What other hints do you have for nurses planning for retirement?

A. Don't pay your house off early if you're under 50, because that interest is tax deductible. This is especially true if you have unsecured debt; get rid of that debt and then work from there.

Q. Any other financial tips?

A. If you want to manage your money, you have to make a budget and follow it. If you're having financial problems, take a 3-month period and write down everything — every dime, every penny, that you spend. It's the only way to know where the money is going.

(continued)

Then once you know where the money is going, you're in a position to make financial decisions.

And be realistic about the decisions. Maybe you really do need that cup of coffee from the coffee shop in the morning. If it's important to you, just budget for it. If you're coming from a place of deprivation that's an extreme, too. The key is to keep everything in balance.

A lawyer speaks: This is general advice and may not apply to your particular situation and shouldn't take the place of common sense or consulting with your own tax professional or financial adviser.

When Is It Time to Move On?

It may not be the prettiest of subjects, but we'd be irresponsible if we didn't address—at least minimally—the question, "When is it time to leave nursing?"

Well, first of all, your answer might be "never." It's entirely possible that you enjoy nursing so much that you plan to keep at it until you slip gently off to the big break room in the sky, or at least until you retire. This was the case for some of the nurses we interviewed, who expressed thoughts such as, "I am not leaving until I retire" (med/surg nurse, RN for 23 years); "I don't think of leaving because I enjoy the nurses and love the patients," (patient educator, RN for 19 years); and "[I would only leave] if there were absolutely no nursing jobs available," (ER nurse, RN for 7 years).

Clearly these nurses, especially those with many years of experience, have found a way to make nursing a sustainable career for themselves. We have picked the brains of these nurses and quoted them throughout this book so that we are all able to benefit from their wisdom. However, you personally have access to many nurses we as authors will never meet. We encourage you to corner the experienced nurses you admire most and interrogate them about how they have managed to survive and maybe even love their life as nurse.

Even with the advice and support of coworkers, helpful resources, trying to advocate for change, and attempting to find a niche within the nursing profession, some RNs will find they are simply not able to continue nursing. If this is the case for you, don't be afraid to save what you might call "freedom money" and search for a better path for yourself. As clinical coordinator and RN Kathryn Cantley says, "If after you've done it for a while you discover your heart is not in it, get out [of nursing] and figure something else out. There is nothing more distressing than having a nurse care for you who clearly doesn't want to be there."

Before you leave, though, explore all your options. Is there another type of nursing you might enjoy more? Could you find a patient population that might be a better fit with your personality? Would an advanced degree or a new role give you a fresh perspective? If you are dealing with injuries, perhaps you can look at what kind of change would make nursing more physically sustainable for you. Molly Raimnodi, who has been an RN for 31 years, explained her situation like this, "I'm not sure [if I've reached my career goals]. I never thought I might not be able to physically do nursing, " but, she adds, "I might possibly transfer to a less physical aspect of nursing."

Finally, whether your goal is to retire as a nurse or only survive until the next paycheck, take inspiration from the responses of your fellow nurses when asked "What keeps you in nursing?"

"Satisfaction that I am doing a worthwhile job and can actually make a difference in the care of a patient."

—Molly Raimnodi

"I love to take care of people…and make a difference in their lives. Even if for an instant I love to make them smile, give them hope…if I were physically not able to work with patients would consider changing careers. But it would have to be one in which I would be helping people."

—DL

"I didn't become a nurse until I was in my late thirties. What keeps me in it is that it offers me so much. It's stimulating and fulfilling and fun. Everything that nurses are supposed to be i.e. nurturing, caring and compassionate has been my experience within nursing. I've always said that nursing has given me much more than I've given to it. "

—Kathryn Cantley

"I am still so passionate about this profession, it would have to be really horrible for me to leave. I would like for us to band and unite for the common good of those we try to heal. But I believe in the mission that we jointly stated at graduation. And I feel that we as healers can change the planet."

—Regina Moore

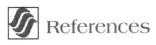 # References

American Association of Colleges of Nursing (April, 2003). Nursing Shortage Fact Sheet. Washington, DC: American Association of Colleges of Nursing.

Bureau of Labor Statistics (November 2001). *Monthly Labor Review.* Washington, DC: Bureau of Labor Statistics.

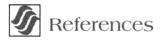 References

1. American Association of Colleges of Nursing. (March, 1999). While demand for RNs climbs, undergraduate nursing enrollments decline. Retrieved June 2000 from the World Wide Web http://www.aacn.nche.edu/Media/Backgrounders/enbk98wb.htm

2. Sigma Theta Tau International Honor Society of Nursing. (June, 1999). Facts about the shortage. Unpublished report: Author.

3. French, E., & Lavendero, R. (1990). *Nursing recruitment & retention: Strategies that work.* Laguna Niguel, CA: American Association of Critical-Care Nurses

4. McKibbin, R.C. (1990). The nursing shortage and the 1990s. Kansas City, MO: American Nurses Association.

5. Foskett, N.H., & Hemsley-Brown, J.V. (March, 1998) Perceptions of nursing as a career among young people in schools and colleges. Southampton, England: Centre for Research in Education Marketing: University of Southampton.

6. Stevens, K., & Walker, Eleanor, E. (January, 1993). Choosing a career: Why not nursing for more high school seniors? *Journal of Nursing Education, 32*(1), 13–17.

7. May, F.E., Champion, V., & Austin, J.K. (September, 1991). Public values and beliefs toward nursing as a career. *Journal of Nursing Education, 30*(7), 303–310.

8. Williams, B., Wertenberger, D.H., & Gushuliak, T. (1997). Why students choose nursing. *Journal of Nursing Education, 36*(7), 346–348.

9. Wilson, C.S., & Mitchell, B.S. (1999). Nursing 2000: Collaboration to promote careers in registered nursing. *Nursing Outlook, 47*(2), 56–61.

10. Kohler, P., & Edwards, T. (January, 1990). High school students' perceptions of nursing as a career choice. *Journal of Nursing Education, 29*(1), 26–30.

Resources

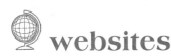 **websites**

American Association of Retired People Financial Future Project
www.aarpfinancialfuture.org/
As you probably already know, you don't have to be retired to use the services of the extremely well-organized AARP. At this site, you can order a free financial planning CD (well, they charge a few bucks for postage) designed for the pre-retiree aged 40 to 60 with limited or no knowledge of personal financial issues. The CD includes interactive exercises as well as case studies. At the AARP main site, you can also read about the rights of older workers and how older workers can best market themselves to employers.

American Nurses Association Online Scholarship Listing
www.nursingsociety.org/career/scholarships_opps.html
If you're considering going back to school, don't let lack of cash get in your way; check out this list of scholarship opportunities.

Department of Labor: Cobra Information Home Page
http://www.dol.gov/dol/topic/health-plans/cobra.htm
If you're thinking about changing jobs but are worried about losing your health insurance, take a quick peek at this site. Explains what COBRA is (hint: they don't mean Ricki Ticki Tavi's arch nemesis) what makes you eligible for it and what you can do if your former employer doesn't cooperate.

Idealist.org
www.idealist.org
It sounds antithetical, but if you're burned out on nursing, you might try doing it for free. You'll find out if it's the working environment, not the profession itself that was tormenting you. Idealist contains information about U.S.- and Canada-based volunteer opportunities and jobs with community-based nonprofits, while Websites such as www.flyinghospital.org, www.operationsmile.org, and www.imva.org have information about volunteer opportunities in other countries.

My Free CE
www.myfreece.com
"Free" is somewhat of a misnomer, but this site does provide very low-cost continuing education. Courses are well written and you can print out CE certificates as soon as you pass the test, which is certainly handy if you

have some kind of CE emergency. Includes comprehensive offerings with courses ranging from how to interpret paps to improving MD-RN interactions.

Nurse-Sponsors

www.nursesponsors.com/registration.html

Nurse-Sponsors organize expos for nurses returning to the workplace. Check out this site to see if they're coming to a city near you!

Silence to Voice

www.silencetovoice.com

This site is the online home of Silence to Voice: What Nurses Know and Must Communicate to the Public. Silence to Voice is a communication guidebook for nurses. The authors (Bernice Buresh and Suzanne Gordon) put the book together with the hopes of providing nurses the tools and inspiration they need to communicate effectively with the public about the role of the professional nurse. The book is quite wide ranging and gives tips about everything from ways of talking about nursing work to friends to how to pitch op-ed pieces to newspapers. You can read excerpts from the book on the site. This book is an important nursing development tool. We should have learned about this in nursing school, but most of us didn't.

Study Abroad

www.studyabroad.com

If you're going back to school anyway, why not take the plunge and schedule a semester to study abroad? At this site, you can search a huge number of programs by both country/region and type of education/subject. You can even book discount airfare. There are a number of nursing programs listed; for example, we found out Michigan State University has a nursing exchange program at King's College in London. C'mon, what are you waiting for, go dust off your passport!

Index